HEALTHY CHILDREN

HEALTHY CHILDREN

How Parents, Teachers, and Community Can Help to Prevent Obesity in Children

Smita Guha

ROWMAN & LITTLEFIELD
Lanham • Boulder • New York • London

Published by Rowman & Littlefield
A wholly owned subsidiary of The Rowman & Littlefield Publishing Group, Inc.
4501 Forbes Boulevard, Suite 200, Lanham, Maryland 20706
www.rowman.com

Unit A, Whitacre Mews, 26-34 Stannary Street, London SE11 4AB

British Library Cataloguing in Publication Information Available

Library of Congress Cataloging-in-Publication Data Available

ISBN: 978-1-4758-2665-4 (cloth: alk. paper)
ISBN: 978-1-4758-2667-8 (electronic)

∞ ™ The paper used in this publication meets the minimum requirements of
American National Standard for Information Sciences—Permanence of Paper for
Printed Library Materials, ANSI/NISO Z39.48-1992.

Printed in the United States of America

This book is dedicated to all the children of the world.

CONTENTS

INTRODUCTION

This book is geared toward educators, teachers, and parents of young children, especially children with health issues. It will be appropriate for scholars, professionals, and policy makers who are involved with children. A typical reader needs no technical background or expertise. I hope to reach a general audience, especially teachers, parents, and school administrators. Further, I hope to reach those in the student audience who are endeavoring to make a change in lifestyle.

Obesity among children is a national and international concern. The focus of the book is to provide evidence-based strategies to assist parents and educators to foster healthy weight gain in children and to empower children to be active agents of change in their own health behavior.

The book will contribute greatly to the literature in the field focusing on national and international concern about childhood obesity and, further, highlighting the problems with obesity prediabetes, type 2 diabetes, etc. Specifically, the book will provide research findings that children who are healthy do better cognitively, socially, emotionally, and, of course, physically. Leading a healthy life helps children live a higher quality of life.

The book will provide a model that can be implemented at home and in school. The model will encompass nutrition education for children. Music will be a significant part in this model that will encourage children to sing and dance to the beat. Dance is a form of exercise that will help children overcome weight issues. Music will be able to heal the children who are socially not accepted by their peers for their weight issues. Team sports and individual sports will be an integral part of the book. Adults involved in the lives of children will be able to follow the model from the book to help the children.

CHAPTER 1: MOTIVATING AND ENGAGING CHILDREN TO BE ACTIVE AGENTS OF THEIR HEALTH BEHAVIOR

This chapter will focus on the following questions and issues: What constitutes health? Why is being healthy important for young children? What factors contribute to staying healthy among children? The chapter will provide a review of research literature in the field, sharing the preexisting models and theories in the field. The emphasis will be on how educators and parents can really effect change in the children they care for. The main focus of this chapter is how to empower children to be active agents of change.

CHAPTER 2: EXPERTS'S OPINIONS AND NUTRITION UNIT

This chapter will focus on developing positive approaches to nutrition education and diet among children through curricular integration. Input from experts such as pediatricians, scientists, dieticians, or nutritionists in the field is provided. This chapter will provide strategies and demonstrate possible ways that teachers can integrate nutritional models across curricula in English, math, science, and social studies.

CHAPTER 3: IMPORTANCE OF PHYSICAL EXERCISE

This chapter will focus on the importance of physical exercise at school, at home, and in the community. Sports, music, and dance will contribute to the aspect of physical exercise among children. Input from experts in the field will be provided. A model will be further developed that will effectively help children get their necessary exercise while having fun with their peers.

CHAPTER 4: SOCIAL AND EMOTIONAL CHALLENGES FOR CHILDREN WITH HEALTH ISSUES

In this chapter, social factors will be highlighted for children who have weight issues. Children with these health issues often suffer from lack of self-esteem, develop a stigma, and/or become victims of bullying. Effective strategies to reduce bullying and help the victim will be provided.

CHAPTER 5: THE ROLES OF FAMILY AND SCHOOL IN PROVIDING NUTRITION EDUCATION FOR CHILDREN

This chapter will focus on the role of the family, especially parents. This chapter will target the family in providing nutrition education for their children. Parents will be encouraged to help their children avoid a sedentary lifestyle, limit time for watching TV and also limit hours on video games and cell phones. Parents will also be educated on the importance of rest and sleep time for their children.

CHAPTER 6: INVOLVEMENT OF THE COMMUNITY IN PROMOTING HEALTHY DEVELOPMENT FOR CHILDREN

This chapter encourages parents and teachers to be involved in the community in promoting overall healthy development for children. Parents learn about dance and sports programs in the community as well as types of food and restaurants in their neighborhood. The author provides strategies to build a partnership with families, schools, and leaders in the community such as medical doctors and community nurses to promote healthy activities for children.

The chapter helps adults focus on the kind of advertisements that have a negative impact on children's decision-making processes with regard to making healthy choices.

CHAPTER 7: STRATEGIES TO WORK COLLABORATIVELY TO PREVENT AN OBESITY EPIDEMIC

This last chapter provides strategies for collaboration among parents, educators, and community leaders for the benefit of children. If children are developing healthy habits, then an obesity epidemic can be prevented. The author suggests strategies as to how educators and parents really affect change in children by providing healthy role models to develop positive behaviors. The focus is on dyadic relationships. Overall healthy children will reflect healthy bodies, minds, and spirits.

ESSENTIAL NEEDS

Almost 14 percent of American children over age six and 12 percent of adolescents are obese. This is more than double the rate thirty years ago. The impact of childhood obesity reaches beyond the individual family and society. However, the epidemic is continuously growing, gaining momentum with each new year.

Over the decades, approaches to obesity treatment and prevention focused on genetics, and explored diets and individual eating behaviors. The focus has since shifted to societal interventions. Although the debate continues over how much influence to assign to heredity and how much to cultural and environmental factors, most adult obesity is rooted in childhood. Current research indicates that a strongly integrated program is the most effective way to success in overcoming obesity.

The World Health Organization (WHO) recently projected that by 2012 in countries like the United States, health-care costs may amount to as much as 17.7 percent of the GDP (gross domestic product). Furthermore, children with obesity issues may be the first generation ever to have a shorter life expectancy than that of their parents. Since children spend most of their time in school and at home, it is important for teachers, school administrators, and parents to help children develop healthy habits to lead a long and healthy life.

GAPS IN KNOWLEDGE

1. How can teachers take a leadership role in promoting health and nutrition among children?
2. How can parents take an active role in ensuring health and nutrition among children?
3. How can teachers and parents partner and collaborate for children's health and nutritional needs to prevent obesity?

4. How can teachers and parents take advantage of the community in promoting health and nutrition among children?
5. How can parents and teachers involve the community to promote health, nutrition, and physical exercise programs for children?
6. How can children be encouraged to take the driver's seat and be responsible for their own health so that they can be healthy throughout their lives?
7. How can parents, teachers, and the community help encourage children to practice healthy living?

Discussion of global perspectives will explore the current state of childhood obesity worldwide and will also focus on future projections and contributing factors associated with childhood obesity, as well as what it means to children, families, and society. Further, recommendations and steps to address and prevent childhood obesity will be discussed.

Although there are a number of diet and weight-loss books on the market, very few focus on the strategies that adults need to take in order to help children with weight issues. To prevent an obesity epidemic, family, school, and community have to work together to pursue effective strategies in a collaborative partnership.

Obesity is fast becoming an epidemic—a national concern—and this book will focus on the role of adults in guiding children in developing healthy eating habits. It will emphasize behavioral factors that impact the eating habits of children and also will involve school and home in providing physical activities for children.

The goal of this book is to assist the audience in finding effective means to promote health and nutrition among children. It is directed at the teachers and parents of children to guide them as partners in promoting health and nutrition among their children. This book will help both teachers and parents to involve the community, and will also encourage adults to help children learn to be responsible for their own health so that they will continue to be healthy throughout their lives.

The idea is to ignite the spark among children so that they are able to realize how important it is to be healthy. Not only will healthy children be able to prevent weight-related disease, they will also have better social lives. Parents and teachers need to realize that children who are healthy do better academically and overall have better lives. This book will provide strategies for adults to help children, focusing on an integrative approach in addressing the obesity pandemic.

I

MOTIVATING AND ENGAGING CHILDREN TO BE ACTIVE AGENTS OF THEIR HEALTH BEHAVIOR

LEARNING OBJECTIVES

1. What constitutes health?
2. Why is being healthy important for young children?
3. What are the concerns of obesity?
4. What are the causes of obesity?
5. Learn about the background of the problem and related research in the field.
6. What factors contribute to staying healthy among children?
7. How can teachers and parents motivate and engage children in caring for their health?

Being physically healthy is a combination of good nutrition, regular exercise, and a sufficient amount of rest. Mental health refers to the cognitive, social, and emotional well-being of a person. The World Health Organization defines mental health as "a state of well-being in which the individual realizes his or her own abilities, can cope with the normal stresses of life, can work productively and fruitfully, and is able to make a contribution to his or her community."

As defined by the Merriam-Webster dictionary, health is the condition of being sound in body, mind, or spirit. According to the World Health Organization, health is defined as "a state of complete physical, mental, and social well-being and not merely the absence of disease or infirmity." There is a wide acceptance that health can be divided into two facets: physical health and mental health.

Being healthy is so important for young children who are growing at such a rapid rate. They need the proper nutrition and exercise in order to maintain a healthy body, mind, and spirit. Proper nutrition and exercise lead to a longer and more enjoyable life. Children can learn healthy habits at a young age and this will definitely benefit them for the years to come.

Leading a healthy lifestyle is important for children to prevent disease and other health complications in adulthood. It is essential to establish healthy eating and regular exercise habits to help children stay healthy throughout their lives. There are many benefits of good nutrition such as strong bones and muscles, good energy levels, increased ability to fight off sickness and disease, faster healing, easier recovery from illness or injury, and reduced risk of health complications in the future and, of course, mental well-being and an increased ability to learn and concentrate. The body has three main uses for nutrients:

- Source of energy
- Materials for growth and maintenance of body tissue
- Regulation of body process

An inadequate supply of nutrients or poor utilization of nutrients may lead to *malnutrition* or *undernutrition* resulting in abnormal body function and general poor health. Malnutrition is a serious problem, especially for infants and young children. Lack of essential nutrients and insufficient calories can be extremely detrimental to their early growth and development and cannot always be reversed with improved dietary intake. At the other end, a diet high in calories and fat and a lack of exercise lead to obesity.

Due to the many benefits of a healthy lifestyle, it is essential to make children active agents in their physical and mental well-being. Children should be educated in making the right decisions for healthy eating as well as have the opportunity to engage in physical activity. Parents are the key people in helping their children choose healthy food options.

DIETARY GUIDELINES

- Eat a variety of foods
- Balance the food you eat with physical activity
- Choose a diet with plenty of grain products, vegetables, and fruits
- Choose a diet low in fat, saturated fat, and cholesterol
- Choose a diet with more fiber
- Choose a diet moderate in sugars
- Choose a diet moderate in salt and sodium
- Servings of vegetables (3–5) and fruit (2–4) are recommended

Parents can help children by offering healthy food options at home while limiting the amount of fast food, takeout food, and junk food. They can educate themselves on food labels and the recommended calorie intake for their children. Parents can also be good role models for their children by eating together as a family and avoiding the use of treats or junk food as rewards. In order to motivate children to be physically active, there are three keys:

1. Choosing the right activities for a child's age
2. Offering kids plenty of opportunity to be active
3. Keeping the focus on fun.

By providing children with the guidance, support, and opportunity to make smart health decisions, parents can help them to become independent agents in a healthy lifestyle.

CONCERNS WITH OBESITY

Childhood obesity has become an enormous problem in the United States. According to the Centers for Disease Control and Prevention, "Childhood obesity has more than doubled in children and quadrupled in adolescents in the past 30 years. The percentage of children aged 6–11 years in the United States who were obese increased from 7% in 1980 to nearly 18% in 2012. Similarly, the percentage of adolescents aged 12–19 years who were obese increased from 5% to nearly 21% over the same period." Clearly the rate of obesity is increasing immensely in a short amount of time.

A poor diet in childhood can lead to major health risks that can cause illness and even death. Obesity can cause adverse effects such as high cholesterol or high blood pressure and symptoms of prediabetes, all of which can result in cardiovascular problems. Obesity can also lead to bone and joint problems, as well as psychological distress for some individuals. Long-term effects of obesity in adults can lead to heart attack and stroke, type 2 diabetes, osteoarthritis, and certain types of cancer. Specifically, childhood obesity can lead to:

1. Type 2 diabetes. Type 2 diabetes is a lifelong (chronic) disease in which there is a high level of sugar (glucose) in the blood. With type 2 diabetes, the body does not make or use insulin well. Insulin is a hormone that helps glucose get into the cells to give them energy. Without insulin, too much glucose stays in the blood. High blood glucose, over time, can lead to serious problems with the heart, eyes, kidneys, nerves, and gums and teeth. Risk of type 2 diabetes increases if the individual is obese, has a family history of diabetes, or

does not exercise. With type 2 diabetes on the rise among children, promoting healthy eating habits from a young age is paramount.

2. Metabolic syndrome. Metabolic syndrome is not a disease itself but rather a cluster of conditions that can put a child at risk for developing heart disease, type 2 diabetes, or other health problems. This group of conditions includes high blood pressure, high blood sugar, high levels of triglycerides (a type of fat) in the blood, low levels of HDL (high-density lipoprotein, often referred as "good" cholesterol), and excess abdominal fat.

3. High cholesterol and high blood pressure. A child can develop high blood pressure or high cholesterol if he or she eats a poor diet. These factors can contribute to the buildup of plaques in the arteries. These plaques can cause arteries to narrow and harden, which can lead to a heart attack or stroke later in life.

4. Asthma. Children who are overweight or obese may be more likely to have asthma.

5. Sleep disorders. Obstructive sleep apnea is a potentially serious disorder in which a child's breathing repeatedly stops and starts when he or she sleeps. It can be a complication of childhood obesity.

6. Nonalcoholic fatty liver disease (NAFLD). This disorder, which usually has few or no symptoms, causes fatty deposits to build up in the liver. NAFLD can lead to scarring and liver damage.

7. Early puberty or menstruation. Being obese can create hormone imbalances that may cause puberty to start earlier than expected.

8. Low self-esteem and becoming a victim of bullying. Children often tease or bully their overweight peers who may suffer a loss of self-esteem and an increased risk of depression as a result.

9. Depression. Low self-esteem can create overwhelming feelings of hopelessness in some overweight children. When children lose hope, they may become depressed. A depressed child may lose interest in normal activities, sleep more than

usual, or cry a lot. Some depressed children hide their sadness and appear "emotionally low" instead.

10. Behavior and learning problems. Overweight children tend to have more anxiety and poorer social skills than normal-weight children have. At one extreme, these problems may lead overweight children to act out and disrupt their classrooms. At the other, they may cause overweight children to socially withdraw.

Source: Mayo Clinic and U.S. National Library of Medicine

WHAT CAUSES OBESITY?

The reason for the obesity epidemic lies in consuming an unhealthy diet. The main problems are foods containing white flour, refined white sugar, and high fructose corn syrup, along with the consumption of soft drinks and fast food (Wayne, 2009). Moreover, certain toxins and chemicals contained in food can cause obesity.

Based on research, eating at "fast-food" restaurants has increased and is linked to obesity. Jeffery et al. (2006) concluded that eating at "fast-food" restaurants can be positively associated with children having a high fat diet and body mass index (BMI). BMI has been reported to be the strongest childhood predictor of adult metabolic syndrome. Other reasons for obesity are lack of exercise and an insufficient amount of sleep time.

The physiological cause for obesity is *metabolic syndrome*, which causes accelerated aging and disease. Metabolic syndrome is a complex health condition that affects an estimated 25 percent of Americans, and most probably a similar percentage around the world. It begins with an inability to manage blood sugar, which creates a state of glucose intolerance or insulin resistance. Insulin resistance contributes to a multitude of conditions including high cholesterol levels, high blood pressure, high blood insulin levels, and obesity.

Child obesity has frequently been linked to the amount of time spent by children watching television or using other electronic devices. Compared to children who watch less than 30 minutes or between 30 and 60 minutes, children watching one to two hours and more than two hours of TV daily had significantly higher BMI z-scores ($p = 0.0002$ and $p < 0.0001$, respectively). Using logistic regression, children who watched more than one hour of TV daily had an odds ratio of 1.521 for overweight and 1.717 for obesity, as compared to those who watched less than one hour daily. In addition, keeping electronic devices in children's bedrooms has also been linked to obesity (Veugelers, 2012).

As these activities are typically taking place within the house, parents should cap the TV viewing time at a maximum of one hour per day, and focus on engaging children in other activities that require greater physical activity and energy expenditure levels, such as dancing, playing soccer, or basketball.

BACKGROUND OF THE PROBLEM

The most recent nationally representative survey data for the years 2003–2006 estimates that 11.3 percent of children and adolescents aged 2 through 19 years residing in the United States are overweight with a BMI greater than or equal to the 97th percentile of the 2000 CDC (Centers for Disease Control and Prevention) BMI-for-age growth charts and 16.3 percent are at or above the 95th percentile. Approximately one-fourth of all toddler and preschool children in the United States are estimated to be overweight or at risk of overweight (Ogden et al., 2008).

Racial/ethnic disparities have been reported from a nationally representative sample of US children at four years of age, with the highest prevalence among Native American/Alaskan Native preschool children for whom obesity is twice as common as in non-Hispanic white or Asian children, with an intermediate prevalence among Hispanic and non-Hispanic black children (Anderson & Whitaker, 2009). Another study, Harnack et al. (2009), indicated a low awareness among parents of the overweight status of their preschool children. Parents of overweight children who do not recognize their child's weight status may be unlikely to engage in obesity prevention efforts.

Approximately one-third of children aged 6 to 11 years (33.3 percent) and adolescents aged 12 to 19 years (34.1 percent) are either at risk of overweight or are overweight. It has been known for some time that weight status tends to track through childhood. By the age of eight years, most children are in the BMI percentile channel that they will follow until the end of growth in late adolescence (Rolland-Cachera et al., 1988).

Taveras et al. (2009) reports that whereas weight-for-length (WFL) at birth was only minimally associated with subsequent overweight, rapid gains in WFL in the first six months of life were associated with sharply increased risk of later obesity. This suggests that early interventions to prevent rapid increase in weight status in the first months of life may help reduce children's risk of obesity later in childhood.

In another study, children who were overweight at thirteen years of age had gained more weight by the age of two or three years than their normal-weight peers. Others have shown that BMI tracks over time from childhood through adolescence and into adulthood (Guo et al., 2002).

At young ages, increases in the prevalence of overweight may be influenced by a shift in eating patterns toward larger portion sizes of energy-dense foods (Lioret et al., 2009). Further, data also indicates that parents may be responsible for feeding patterns and eating habits introduced very early in life that may last a lifetime, with serious health consequences (Ziegler et al., 2006).

A study from Israel (Shibli et al., 2008) indicates evidence of increased health risk in overweight infants and toddlers (less than or equal to two years of age; weight-for-length greater than or equal to 95th percentile). An imbalance between excess dietary energy intake and inadequate energy expenditure are ultimately the determinants of overweight status.

A study from Australia reports that being overweight at five years of age was associated with BMI and overweight status of young adults at twenty-one years of age (Mamun et al., 2009). The importance of the tracking phenomenon for overweight lies in the well-established knowledge that increased body weight in adulthood is highly associated with increased health risks.

Patterns of physical activity and inactivity may begin to be established at an early age in the home environment. When combined with a diet of highly energy-dense foods, patterns of inactivity may help to explain the increasing prevalence of overweight among young children.

In early childhood the home environment may be crucial in establishing the framework for reinforcement of knowledge or practices consistent with energy balance. There is evidence that children who remain home with their parents during the preschool years are less likely to be obese than children cared for by other family, friends, or neighbors, indicating that there may be a need for a larger parental role with regard to the management of their children when they are away from home (Maher et al., 2008).

In addition to diet and activity, sleep patterns influence the development of children. For example a study reported that daily sleep duration of less than 12 hours during infancy appears to be a risk factor for being overweight among preschool-aged children. Parental social stress, time limitations, work responsibilities, and absence are other factors that may strain parent/child interactions.

THEORETICAL AND RESEARCH PERSPECTIVE

According to literature, "nutritionists, social scientists, and educators are able to demonstrate a positive correlation between proper nutrition and intellectual functioning resulting in improved learning" (Cosgrove, 1991). A child who is well-nourished will be active. A child who is active learns more. As Cosgrove (1991) mentions, "Healthy, well-nourished children benefit more from formal education than undernourished children." Therefore, children need to be educated about proper nutrition. Nutrition education is the process of helping children develop the knowledge, skills, and motivation needed to make appropriate food choices.

During the early childhood years, when children are in their "absorbent mind" (Montessori, 1965), nutrition education should begin. As (Cosgrove, 1991) mentions: "Particularly during the early years when children are both an impressionable and captive audience, and when habits are formed, nutrition education is critical to the formation of health promoting nutritional concepts and behaviors. It is during these early years that nutrition education is most successful."

Piaget indicates that children imitate adults, therefore, "adults must be mindful of the nutrient needs of children and must use this knowledge in shaping children's food preferences and patterns" (Fuhr & Barclay, 1998). Experience and studies conducted in preschools have shown that, even in these early years, children can be led beyond the names and tastes of foods to an understanding of basic concepts of nutritive value, nutrient function, and the impact of nutrition on health (Swadener & Lubeck, 1995).

As Cosgrove (1991) mentions, "by cooking in the classroom with young children, you can begin to open the door to good nutrition and positive well-being. Many kinds of learning are involved in cooking; motor, sensory, conceptual and social skills all play an important part in food preparation. All five senses are involved."

Since children spend a lot of time at school, school should take an active role in nutrition education among children. Breakfast and lunch times can be instructional periods that afford teachers many opportunities to structure a learning environment that promotes food and nutrition education, social interaction, development of concepts and skills, and self-directed activities that allow children to make choices. Young children should have a variety of experiences and opportunities that provide understanding of nutrition for their personal health (Seefeldt & Galper, 2002).

Children at an early age may not have an idea of healthy food. Thus, as Seefeldt and Galper (2002) mention: "Teachers should be aware of the concepts and the misconceptions they (children) have about health. Further, children do not necessarily understand that some foods are nutritionally better than others."

Young children need to become individuals who have a lifelong responsibility for their own health and personal care, including dental hygiene, cleanliness, and exercise. Some early childhood educators have noticed that despite recommendations for good nutrition, changing family styles are having an adverse impact on the nutritional habits of many young children.

More sugar and fats now enter their diets, and many cooking activities suggested for the classroom use do not include nutritional learning objectives. Thus, parents and teachers should be committed to the premise that the care and nourishment of the human body is essential to the healthy development of the children (Seefeldt & Galper, 2002).

Teachers must understand the influence that family has over children; to ensure maximum influence on the health and well-being of young children, adults must consider the influences that shape the food preferences and eating patterns of young children. Family is the single most important influence on what young children eat.

To maintain school-home continuity, nutrition education information needs to be provided to family members about the availability and importance of nutritious meals inside and outside of school; children receiving a nutritional meal at home are more likely to develop good eating patterns. Since each family's culture affects a child's food preferences and eating routines, caregivers and teachers should work with families to establish a mutual understanding of each child's nutritional needs and how those needs can be met.

However, few teachers attempt to integrate nutrition education into their daily curriculum. Cosgrove (1991) mentions, "Total commitment from parents is a crucial part of any nutrition program." Head Start has emphasized, since its inception, that respecting family food preferences and eating patterns, while providing nutrition education, is critical to the development of sound nutritional concepts and behaviors.

Many Americans seem to be oblivious or unconvinced by scientific research that suggest that "personal choices" may not account for all cases of obesity. According to Jou (2014), the majority of Americans believe that obesity is caused due to overeating and/or the lack of exercising. He cited that the German pathologist Carl Von Noorden described two types of obesity: exogenous and endogenous. Some people are prone to obesity and endogenous obesity should not be dismissed.

"School-based interventions have also been highlighted in numerous reports as one of several settings needing investment and resources to control the obesity epidemic." This study found that "parents with overweight children did not recognize when their child was overweight nor feel concerned about their weight." The child's home is likely to have the greatest influence on a child's eating and physical activity behaviors. Supportive school interventions can only reinforce and complement any effort to prevent obesity that happens at home (Sutherland, Gill, & Binns, 2004).

Schools have an important role in helping children and their families develop healthy eating habits. To the children, teachers are role models and for the families, teachers are a resource. Teachers need to take the initiative in building awareness about proper diet and in providing opportunities for exercise.

MOTIVATING AND ENGAGING CHILDREN TO BE HEALTHY: ROLE OF ADULTS

The best way to motivate children to be active agents of healthy behavior is by being an active participant in demonstrating healthy eating habits. Children learn by observing; therefore, adults can provide a positive model, consistently sitting together with the children during meal time without any distractions and eating the same foods.

Children feel encouraged to eat what others are eating as well. Teachers and parents can also link positive connotations to healthy food items such as "Mmm, carrots taste good!" or "I love carrots!" while eating carrots. Adults can also teach children the benefits of healthy food choices and encourage children to participate in helping out in the kitchen. Children can complete fun activities that include healthy choices in preparing food by following a new recipe.

Teaching children what unhealthy food choices can do to their bodies further reinforces the idea that they should avoid things that can be detrimental to their health. They must also be encouraged to be active. Exposing children to a positive, social, and loving environment promotes a successful and healthy lifestyle.

Parents have the biggest role to play in helping their children along the road to healthier living. Making mealtimes playful can promote healthier eating habits for your kids. For example, create a food collage: use broccoli florets for trees, carrots and celery for flowers, cauliflower for clouds, and a yellow squash for a sun.

Addressing weight problems in children requires a coordinated plan of physical activity and healthy nutrition. The goal should be to slow or halt weight gain, thereby allowing your child to grow into an ideal weight. Children can go food shopping with their parents; they can be in charge. Let them see all the different fruits and vegetables and have them pick out new ones to try. Emphasis must be placed on the types of food available to children, especially at breakfast, the most important meal of the day.

Children who eat breakfast are generally in better health overall, a fact that may be attributed to the types of food often associated with the morning meal. Breakfast provides a golden opportunity to fortify your children with nutrients. Fiber can help with weight control and has also been linked to lower cholesterol levels. Most brands of cereal contain a large amount of fiber.

A healthy diet and daily physical activity will not only promote a long and healthy life span but also helps achieve academic success. At the early stages of life, children's physical development is crucial and diet plays a large role. It's important to support the link between healthy eating at school, home, and in all other environments.

By educating your child on what is good for their overall health—including their bones, skin, heart, and teeth—they will become more active agents of healthy behavior. Planning, shopping, and cooking meals together are great ways to engage children. Providing opportunities for children is important as they learn through experiences such as cooking in the kitchen with their family members.

Parents are able to motivate children by giving them choices. When children are allowed to pick out their own healthy food items at the supermarket, they become more inclined to understand their own eating habits. Children can help cook or prepare their meals to keep them engaged in learning about healthy eating habits. This process helps motivate children to be powerful and spread their knowledge to their peers.

When parents and children work together as a team, they influence one another to be conscious of what they eat. Families should strive to have family meals each night so that they get an opportunity to discuss all of the healthy food they eat and what nutrients they provide to their bodies. Some important ways to help motivate and engage children to be active agents of healthy behavior are by involving them in physical activities such as sports (soccer, basketball, tennis, swimming, running, etc.), dance (ballet, tap, jazz, gymnastics), and any other activities that involve movement.

Eating good food and having an active lifestyle help to promote confidence, structure, and flexibility; together they will also strengthen the child's body and immune system. Parents need to teach their children the fun part of exercise. Especially with young children, parents can compare them to "strong superheroes." What is most important is to keep children active and motivated.

DISCUSSION QUESTIONS

1. What constitutes health?
2. Why is being healthy important for young children?
3. What are the concerns of obesity?
4. What are the causes of obesity?
5. What factors contribute to sustaining health among children?
6. How can teachers and parents motivate and engage children in caring for their health?
7. What are the main ideas contained in this chapter?
8. Measure yourself by comparing your habits with the eating and socializing aspects of this chapter.

REFERENCES

Anderson, S. E., and R. C. Whitaker. 2009. Prevalence of obesity among US preschool children in different racial and ethnic groups. *Archives of Pediatrics & Adolescent Medicine* 163: 344–48.

Cosgrove, M. S. 1991. Cooking in the classroom: The doorway to nutrition. *Young Children* 46 (3): 43–46.

Fuhr, J .E., & K. H. Barclay. 1998. The importance of appropriate nutrition and nutrition education. *Young Children* 53 (1) (January): 74–80.

Guo, S. S., W. Wu, W. C. Chumlea, and A. F. Roche. 2002. Predicting overweight and obesity in adulthood from body mass index values in childhood and adolescence. *American Journal of Clinical Nutrition* 76 (3) (September): 653–58.

Harnack, L., L. Lytle, J. H. Himes, M. Story, G. Taylor, and D. Bishop. 2009. Low awareness of overweight status among parents of preschool-aged children, Minnesota, 2004–2005. *Preventing Chronic Disease* 6: A47.

Jou, C. 2014. The biology and genetics of obesity—A century of inquiries. *New England Journal of Medicine* 370:1874–77.

Jeffery, R. W., J. Baxter, M. McGuire, and J. Linde. 2006. Are fast food restaurants an environmental risk factor for obesity? *International Journal of Behavioral Nutrition and Physical Activity* 3 (2) (January): 1.

Lioret, S., J. L. Volatier, L. Lafay, M. Touvier, and B. Maire. 2009. Is food portion size a risk factor of childhood overweight? *European Journal of Clinical Nutrition* 63: 382–91.

Maher, E. J., G. Li, L. Carter, and D. B. Johnson. 2008. Preschool child care participation and obesity at the start of kindergarten. *Pediatrics* 122: 322–30.

Mamun, A. A., M. J. O'Callaghan, and S. M. Cramb. 2009. Childhood behavioral problems predict young adults' BMI and obesity: Evidence from a birth cohort study. *Obesity* 17 (4) (April).

Montessori, M. 1965. *The Montessori method; Spontaneous activity in education; The Monkssori elementary material.* Cambridge, MA: Robert Bentley.

Ogden, C. L., M. D. Carroll, and K. M. Flegal. 2008. High body mass index for age among US children and adolescents, 2003–2006. *JAMA* 299: 2401–5.

Piaget, J. 1970. In *Carmichael's manual of child psychology*, vol. 1, ed. P. H. Mussen. New York: Wiley.

Rolland-Cachera, M. F., M. Deheeger, F. Pequignot, M. Guilloud-Bataille, F. Vinit, and F. Bellisle. 1988. Adiposity and food intake in young children: The environmental challenge to individual susceptibility. *British Medical Journal (Clinical Research Ed.)* 296: 1037–38.

Seefeldt, C., and A. Galper. 2002. *Active experiences for active children: Science.* Upper Saddle River, NJ: Pearson Education.

Shibli, R., L. Rubin, H. Akons, and R. Shaoul. 2008. Morbidity of overweight (> or = 85th percentile) in the first 2 years of life. *Pediatrics* 122: 267–72.

Sutherland, R., T. Gill, and C. Binns. 2004. Do parents, teachers and health professionals support school-based obesity prevention? *Nutrition & Dietetics* 61 (3): 137–44.

Swadener, B. B., and S. Lubeck, eds. 1995. *Children and Families "At Promise": Deconstructing the Discourse of Risk*. New York: State University of New York Press.

Taveras, E. M., S. L. Rifas-Shiman, M. B. Belfort, K. P. Kleinman, E. Oken, and M. W. Gillman. 2009. Weight status in the first 6 months of life and obesity at 3 years of age. *Pediatrics* 123: 1177–83.

Veugelers, Paul. 2012. Take the TV out of your children's bedroom so they can sleep properly, say researchers. *Daily Mail*, October 23. http://www.dailymail.co.uk/sciencetech/article-2221822/Take-TV-childrens-bedroom-sleep-properly-say-researchers.html.

Wayne, Michael. 2009. Obesity around the world. *Dr. Michael Wayne*, November 17. http://drmichaelwayne.com/blog/obesity-around-the-world/.

Ziegler, P., R. Briefel, N. Clusen, and B. Devaney. 2006. Feeding infants and toddlers study (FITS): Development of the FITS survey in comparison to other dietary survey methods. *Journal of American Dietary Association* 106 (1 Suppl 1) (January): S12–27.

EXPERTS' COMMENTS AND NUTRITION UNIT

LEARNING OBJECTIVES

1. What are some of the experts' comments on preventing obesity among young children?
2. What are some of the suggestions from research in the field with regard to promoting health and nutrition education among young children and preventing obesity?
3. With nutrition as a unit of study, how can teachers teach across curricula (English, math, science, and social studies)?

EXPERTS' COMMENTS ON PREVENTING OBESITY AMONG YOUNG CHILDREN

A medical doctor and a researcher working in an obesity clinic, a nutritionist, a scientist working in the food administration department, and two pediatricians are interviewed.

A doctor and a researcher working in an obesity center note that obesity starts in the home environment with the family's dietary habits. Adults are role models and, therefore, it is a good practice for them to offer healthy food to children in daycare, preschool, and school. Further, they point out that children's menu items in restaurants are mostly white and yellow foods. Adults should encourage children to move away from white and yellow and focus on green. This is because white and yellow colors symbolize fattening, unhealthy food, whereas green represents vegetables.

Similarly, a scientist working in the food administration states that, in general, a healthy diet, exercise, and enough sleep are essential for the prevention of obesity among young children. The rate of obesity increases because of an unhealthy diet. Parents and teachers should provide proper diets to the children in their care.

A nutritionist would like to reinforce healthy eating habits and increase physical activity among children to combat obesity. She suggests having a registered dietitian available in public schools to perform screening for obesity and to ensure that appropriate intervention measures are in place to prevent excessive calorie intake; she also recommends modifying the contents of school vending machines to limit high fat/sugary snacks and to offer children healthy snack choices.

A pediatrician offers a prescription for healthy living outlined in Table 2.1. Another pediatrician recommends three ways to prevent obesity among young children:

- nutrition
- exercise
- behavioral modification

According pediatricians, the most effective way to measure overweight or obesity is by body mass index or BMI. If the child's BMI is 85 to 94 percent, then the child is diagnosed as overweight. If the child's BMI is above 95 percent, then the child is obese; above 99 percent, the child is morbidly obese.

Table 2.1. 8-7-6-5-4-3-2-1-0 Prescription for Healthy Living

8	8–11 hours of sleep each night
7	7 breakfasts every week
6	6 home-cooked meals around the table every week
5	5 servings of fruit and vegetables every day
4	4 positive self-messages every day
3	3 servings of low-fat dairy daily
2	2 hours or less of screen time daily
1	1 hour or more of physical activity daily
0	0 sugar-sweetened beverages per day

From Tucker, J., Eisenmann, J., Howard, K., et al. FitKids360: design, conduct, and outcomes of a Stage 2 pediatric obesity program. *J Obes* 2014; 2014: 37404.

EXPERTS' RECOMMENDATIONS FOR CHILDREN

According to the doctor and researcher, young children have no control of their food intake. It is adults who have to help children maintain a balanced diet. Later on as the children grow up, they have the power to make food choices. Habits are generally formed early in life and it becomes very difficult to change if good habits are not developed in the early childhood years.

The scientist suggests that foods that are low fat, low sugar, and high fiber should be provided to children. Daily exercise also plays a vital part.

The pediatrician feels that a nonpharmacological approach is best. Medicine and/or diet pills are not needed. She makes three recommendations:

1. Nutrition: Eat healthy meals
2. Limit sugar beverages
3. Increase fruit and vegetable consumption, decrease snacks (unless they are healthy snacks such as carrots, cucumbers, etc.), and cut down portion size

For a weight loss or obese diet, she recommends losing less than half a kilogram or about one pound per week in terms of weight. In terms of physical exercise, it is important to increase the duration of unstructured free play. For older children, increase unstructured or structured play—encourage them to participate in sports that they enjoy, like soccer, basketball, or running. For very young children up to four years of age, 180 minutes of any intense physical activity daily is suitable, and for children five years or older, 60 minutes of moderate to rigorous physical activity is ideal. Further, she recommends that adults limit children's screen time to less than two hours per day.

The pediatrician stresses that the focus on a behavioral approach in support of physical activity and a healthy lifestyle must be increased. The family can make a trip to the grocery store and play a game in which each person picks a green vegetable. The family can participate in activities together—throwing and catching a ball, jumping on the trampoline, cycling, or hiking. Families can also decrease the frequency of eating in restaurants and increase the frequency of eating meals together at home. It is also wise to promote self-monitoring; use of food as a reward should be discouraged.

The pediatrician advises that the best way to solve the problem is to have the family create a plan together and make it work. For example, involve the family by asking each family member to pick one green vegetable, one yellow vegetable, and one red vegetable each day and then eat the selected vegetables.

The nutritionist recommends packing a healthy lunch/snack to take outside and staying active throughout the day. Snacks should contain less than 10 grams of sugar, at least 2 grams of fiber, and less than 2 grams of saturated fat per serving. She also strongly believes in limiting electronics/TV to one hour per day.

EXPERTS' RECOMMENDATIONS FOR PARENTS

The doctor and researcher recommend that parents should provide nutritious food. Adults should provide whole grains, vegetables, fruits, and small portions of meat and fish every week. Enjoy eating together as a family. It is also a good idea to have children be in the company of other children who eat healthy meals.

Similarly, the scientist states that healthy food habits start at home. Parents should make a routine for their children. Only healthy food should be kept at home. It is normal for children to ask for junk food because it tastes good, but parents need to be strict and should not allow children to eat unhealthy food.

Healthy food can also be tasty—it is all in how it is prepared. Parents have to make a deal with children who are picky eaters. Parents have to substitute healthy food. As role models, parents should eat healthy foods to show their children what types of foods need to be eaten.

The pediatrician says that the most important recommendations for parents are to ensure at least one hour of physical activity, to eat breakfast together, and to cut down or decrease portion size. Talk to the primary care provider or pediatrician and monitor BMI at regular intervals. Facilitate early intervention to ensure healthy levels of cholesterol, blood sugar, and blood pressure and to monitor diet and daily exercise. Counseling for pregnant mothers is needed regarding adequate nutrition, noting that one of the benefits of nursing or breast-feeding is a decreased chance that the child will become obese.

It is important to support social marketing that promotes healthy food to growing children. The school community should ensure adequate physical education, develop fundamental movement skills, and insist on having recess periods in every school. Further, school should mandate nutritional food at school and in vending machines. The school should include a nutrition education curriculum to promote healthy eating and foster positive image. School should ensure accessibility of play spaces.

Communities need recreational parks and safe walking and hiking routes in residential areas. People need access to improved mental health services and more comprehensive community programs that promote healthy lifestyles, especially among children from low socioeconomic backgrounds, should be established. She firmly believes that there should be a public policy to ensure adequate funding for treatment of obesity and obesity-related comorbidity.

Parents should encourage social marketing of healthy food options and restrict marketing of unhealthy food to young children. Additional incentives could be established to provide more fruits and vegetables at affordable prices.

The nutritionist suggests that parents stock their refrigerators with fresh fruits and vegetables. She advises them not to purchase soft drinks that are filled with sugar. Parents should encourage intake of low-fat milk and other good sources of daily calcium and offer whole-grain, nonsugary cereals for breakfast.

The pediatrician's advice to the parents is to let young children feed themselves; parents often overfeed the child. Families should eat meals together and should show children how to make the right kinds of food choices. Adults in the family should be role models to the children. If parents have long working hours, they need to ensure that children in daycare or after-school programs have structured and nonstructured play or dance activities to improve weight management.

EXPLANATION AND RECOMMENDATION OF THE QUALITY OF DIET FOR CHILDREN

The doctor and researcher suggest that parents need to make healthy food choices easily available to the children. For example, the researcher suggests washing and cutting fresh cauliflower and keeping it in a big container in the refrigerator. Easy accessibility is the key here because if packaged food is easily accessible, then children will reach for that.

Once in a while it is okay to eat any desired food. Too much restriction can increase desire so much that it will lead children to eat a lot of unhealthy food. If the child loses self-control, parents will have to monitor the child more closely. The problem starts when unhealthy food is eaten on a daily basis.

According to the scientist, focus should be on plant-based foods. For nonvegetarian items, choose lean meat, fish, and eggs and avoid red meat. Encourage children to drink a lot of water.

Dietary fiber is an essential constituent of a healthy diet. A research scientist notes that "High-fiber food and fiber supplements are important parts of the public health strategy to overcome the epidemic of chronic diseases such as inflammatory bowel disease, colon cancer, obesity, diabetes and cardiovascular disease" (Yadav et al., 2005). High-fiber foods include vegetables and fruits and should be consumed by everyone.

He mentioned that there are two kinds of fiber: water soluble and water insoluble fiber. Both kinds come from plant cell walls. Both kinds are beneficial to human beings. However, lots of foods we normally eat are not from the plant cell wall. We usually throw away apple and orange skins. However, these outer layers are rich in nutraceuticals and polyphenol. These components are essential in preventing obesity, type 2 diabetes, and heart attacks. Apple skin is also rich in fiber. Parents should wash the apple with warm water and offer the whole apple with skin to the children. Orange juice with pulp is also rich in fiber. We generally throw away orange skin that is rich in fiber, therefore, scientists are trying to dry the orange peel and make it into a powdered form to mix in drinks, milk, and salad dressings.

Other vegetables that are good sources of fiber are green beans, broccoli, cauliflower, and spinach. Further, processed grain by-products like corn fiber, wheat, bran, and barley are good for health. Whole-wheat bread and multigrain bread are healthier than white bread, which has a starchy part. The outer layers in the grains are rich in fiber. He further describes the benefits of fiber:

> Fiber [has fewer] calories. Fiber is not digested in [the] small intestine. It goes to the large intestine and then gets fermented and that generates short chains of fatty acids and forms good bacteria.

1. Water insoluble fiber holds a lot of water. It also absorbs water and increases volume. Since it absorbs water, it helps to excrete the remains. Stool then becomes soft and bowel movement is fast, thereby preventing disease.
2. Soluble fiber has a compound rich in antioxidants. The human body produces toxins. Those toxins produced by [the] oxidation process damage body cells, for example, DNA could get damaged too. The fiber supplies antioxidants that prevent toxic compounds. For example, aurveydic components prevent toxins. All kinds of berries like strawberries and blueberries are rich in antioxidants. Red grapes also have more antioxidants than green grapes.
3. Some fibers have big molecules. Our body hydrolyses to small molecules. They are easily fermented in the small intestine. Those are carbohydrates and are called probiotics. Probiotics are good bacteria, especially good for colon health and prevent[ing] colon cancer. Those probiotics could be received from fiber.

Agriculture residue isolated from sweet grass is called miscanthus. Currently, scientists are making water soluble fiber. On the labels of various foods, such as dairy products and salad dressings, parents should also look for "cellulose derivatives." Gum arabic is a good stabilizer found in canned juice or orange juice.

The nutritionist recommends whole-grain foods: At least half (3 ounces) of the grains eaten daily should be whole grains. On food labels, a whole grain (such as whole wheat, brown rice, or whole oats) should be the first ingredient on the ingredients list.

Focus on calcium-rich foods. Children should drink 2 to 3 cups of fat-free or low-fat milk or eat the equivalent amount of low-fat yogurt and/or cheese every day.

Next on the list are fruits. Aim for 1 1/2 to 2 cups of fruits daily. Choose fruits that are fresh, frozen, canned, or dried. One cup of 100 percent fruit juice is equivalent to one cup of fruit.

Vegetables: Aim for at least 1 1/2 cups of a variety of vegetables daily. Include dark-green vegetables (such as spinach, broccoli, and kale) and orange vegetables (such as carrots, sweet potatoes, and pumpkin).

Lean meats and poultry: Adults should choose lean cuts of meat and poultry prepared without additional fat or oil (for example, baked, broiled, or grilled).

The pediatrician recommends that children should eat a healthy diet, and increase fruits, vegetables, and whole grain consumption. Children should be taking in more calcium and vitamins and less refined sugar and saturated fat. Fiber intake should be increased. Convenience foods such as prepackaged foods or snacks, fast food, restaurant food, sweetened juice, soda, and sports drinks are not healthy and should not be consumed.

For children who are having health issues, implement a healthy diet. The child needs to have the right kind of food. A low-fat, high-carbohydrate diet with a low glycemic index, which incorporates such foods as oatmeal, low-fat yogurt, and barley, is good for children. The "traffic light" or "stoplight" diet—an eating plan that marks green foods, yellow foods, and red foods—has been used for preschool children with good outcomes.

- Green foods: Anybody can eat these; they are low-calorie, high-fiber; consume in unlimited quantities.

- Yellow foods: These foods must be limited in their daily intake as they provide increased nutrients.
- Red foods: These foods are high in fat or simple sugar and should be taken infrequently and not every day. Limit carbohydrate and fat in diet.

However, children can have a protein-bearing modified diet, with a protein intake of 1.5 to 2.5 per kilograms or 3 to 5 pounds per day, 1.5 liters or 6–8 cups of water, 600–900 calories per day.

HEALTH PROBLEMS CAUSED BY OBESITY

The problems that result due to obesity are type 2 diabetes, hypertension, polycystic ovary syndrome, nonalcoholic fatty liver disease, obstructive apnea, orthopedic complications, high blood pressure, high cholesterol or hyperlipidemia, high liver function abnormality, cardiovascular disease, and hepatic steatosis or fatty liver with inflammation and damage.

Other health problems caused by obesity include menstrual irregularity, severe acne, and temporary hair loss or baldness. Acanthosis nigricans, a cutaneous marker of insulin resistance, is also very common. Other problems are gallstones, snoring, sleep apnea, and insulin resistance.

TIPS GIVEN BY EXPERTS IN TERMS OF MOTIVATING CHILDREN TO EAT HEALTHY FOODS

The doctor and the researcher think adults have to keep trying every now and then to feed healthy foods to children. If the children do not like the specific food, adults should temporarily let it go to avoid confrontation. After some time, try again; eventually the child will listen.

The pediatrician believes that first of all, adults need to be good role models. Families need to eat healthy foods, exercise every day, and cultivate good habits. Adults should keep things fun and positive. Children need positive reinforcement and appreciation. It is a good idea to praise children for a job well done. Help children to develop good self-image. It is important to take small steps and gradually change the diet. As a reward, children should not be given candy or sweetened food or video games.

Eat together as a family. Enjoy hearing from your children. It is important to involve children in planning and cooking a meal together. The family will spend quality time together which is an added bonus. Another way is to go to the grocery store together as a family and make a game. Read the label and then involve everyone in a discussion about it. Children will learn how to select the food after reading the label.

The nutritionist suggests that one form of counseling for weight management is motivational interviewing. Through this process, the child can view the current behavior and set up the desired goal. Together with the child, family members take part. Once the child and family have made self-motivational statements, the counselor can help to bring about behavioral change through reflective listening and commentary. This type of interviewing may also help resistant or unmotivated families consider lifestyle changes.

A counselor should talk to children about the food they are eating. Let the child talk about his or her diet and favorite foods. Listen to the child, then praise the child for what the child is doing well. Then explain and try self-motivational treatment. An adult can explain to the child about healthy diet. Further, explain that it is unwise to eat fatty foods because they may create a heart problem. An adult working with a child who has a weight issue can follow three steps:

1. Problem recognition: Identify the child's concern. For example, "you are getting easily tired."

2. Intention: Plan to change diet and lifestyle.
3. Optimism: Encourage the child by suggesting a pleasant activity. For example, the family could go for a walk together for about 30 minutes.

EXPERTS' COMMENTS ON THE IMPORTANCE OF PHYSICAL EXERCISE FOR CHILDREN

The scientist feels strongly that exercise is very important for young children. Exercise helps increase circulation, reduces blood sugar, and stabilizes blood pressure. Children should exercise for at least a couple of hours.

Similar to the scientist, the pediatrician feels strongly that children need to be active every day for healthy growth and development. Children who develop a healthy lifestyle pattern at a young age will carry the benefit the rest of their lives. Further, physical activity promotes better self-esteem. Children should be told that by eating healthy foods, they will develop strong bones, muscles, joints, and heart. That way, children can stay healthy and they will have better social interaction with friends.

Most importantly, parents need to be aware that regular exercise can foster better concentration in school. Physical exercise helps in circulation; children will be more energetic and less tired.

The nutritionist feels that exercise helps prevent excessive weight gain. When calories are taken in excess and/or not expended as energy, the unused calories accumulate as body fat. Exercising may create a caloric deficit that takes fat away. Exercise also makes you feel more energetic.

The pediatrician also feels very strongly that exercise is vital and that the family lifestyle should be changed to accommodate it, if need be. The idea is to have less TV time and less time on the iPad or iPhone. The goal is to have children move away from a sedentary lifestyle. Thirty percent of the time outside of school, children need to play or get involved in heavy exercise like swimming, baseball, or basketball, three days a week or a half hour every day. A pedometer can be used to measure the number of steps taken and to calculate how much more exercise is needed.

Children should not get involved in too many organized activities. Due to lack of time, parents have difficulty in finding the opportunity to cook, and children end up eating snacks and fast food. When families have little time for food preparation, meals are not structured or are rushed in order to accommodate busy lifestyles. During mealtime, food should be eaten slowly and not rushed.

Parents who work long hours have limited time to engage with their children during meals or in exercising together. The family has to make a decision and set up priorities about activities.

According to the pediatricians, the most significant aspect of childhood obesity is the adiposity rebound. The body mass index of children, as a measure of adiposity, increases rapidly during the first five years of life, and then declines around five to six years of age when a child's growth is reduced. That is the time parents have to be especially careful about children's health.

Not only food habits but also parent and child behavioral modification need to be considered. The child care provider should never reward a child with food. Juice is restricted because it has a lot of sugar and as a result the child becomes hungrier. The child needs healthy protein, such as egg whites, chicken, and turkey.

TYPE OF EXERCISE IN PREVENTION OF OBESITY AMONG CHILDREN

The pediatrician recommends physical activity for at least one hour every day. The scientist suggests that children and parents can get involved in exercise together. Further, parents could organize a group consisting of parents and children to get involved in exercise.

Gardening could be a good activity for both children and parents to be active together.

TIPS IN MOTIVATING CHILDREN TO EXERCISE

The doctor and the researcher feel that for children, play should be their exercise. Children should have a lot of fun while playing. They should run around, dribble a ball, and jump, etc. Movement is important for their metabolic health. Parents can start different play sports at home. Parents need to be active so that their children are active.

The pediatrician thinks that children should have the opportunity of both structured and unstructured play. Structured play includes traditional sports like soccer and basketball that children enjoy. Children should choose the sport that they like through trial and error. Family game time can also be very effective. Children should be discouraged from long hours of screen time. Continuous chatting or texting on the phone or spending long hours of watching TV or playing video games is detrimental to the healthy development of children.

If the grocery store is within walking distance, the family can go grocery shopping by walking, and children could be given an incentive by inviting a friend to join them. Children should be encouraged to climb stairs in the shopping mall. Exercise should not be regarded as a reward or a punishment; it is part of daily life. The nutritionist suggests parents enroll their children in various sports programs, get them to walk the dog, ride their bikes, etc.

RESOURCES FOR CHILDREN THAT FAMILIES AND SCHOOLS SHOULD BE AWARE OF

The doctor and the researcher feel that children should play during school at recess on the playground or in a gym. During after-school hours, children can get involved in different school activities and team sports. There are different clubs and teams where children can get involved. If children have no time during weekdays, then more activities should be planned for weekends and on vacations. However, consistency is important to get the best result.

The pediatrician strongly believes that healthy food must be served in school. Only healthy snacks should be made available. Usually, school food tends to be very high in total and saturated fat. If children get hungry faster, they should eat protein. Almost all the schools have vending machines but very few sell low-fat yogurt, fruits, or vegetables.

At the school level, changes need to be made regarding prevention of obesity. Children should engage in different forms of exercise. Two main factors that counselors should focus on are increasing physical activity and improving eating habits through nutrition education. Since children stay in school 60 percent of the time, schools should offer aerobics three times a week. Counselors need to devote more time to discussing nutrition and exercise. They need to look at the family issues and work with the children.

Further, the doctor and the researcher think getting enough sleep is essential for children. Children cannot learn properly or perform well in school if they are tired. There is a strong link between lack of sleep and obesity.

The community should provide healthier choices of food for children. Restaurants should offer healthy food items such as those in the adult menu but in smaller portions for children. Fast-food eating should be replaced by healthy eating with more emphasis on fruits and vegetables.

Parents can take their children to the grocery store and ask them to pick a vegetable and a fruit that they like. If children choose the fruit and the vegetable, there is a greater chance that they will eat these selections. Children should not be afraid to try new food items.

For example, offer carrots, broccoli, cauliflower, green beans, colored peppers, and snap peas, and tell the children to choose any three of their liking. They can snack on these vegetables while waiting for dinner. Also provide whole-grain cereal. If children want to have sugar cereal, then you can mix and match cereal (mix Mini-Wheats with shredded wheat), thereby reducing the sugar content of cereal and doubling the fiber amount.

If the children do not like something, adults can say "OK, try one and give the rest to the others." Adults should act more like facilitators. Broccoli could be roasted or stir-fried to become brighter green. If the food becomes mushy then it does not look good; children may not like to eat it. In fact, overcooked food lacks good nutrition. A small amount of fat is good for children. Salad with olive oil and vinegar is healthy. Another tip is to follow a traditional diet. Children may like to have experiences with spices; herbs used in foods, such as garlic powder or nutmeg in squash, can be inviting. For example, cinnamon in oatmeal gives a nice flavor.

Often parents say that they do not have enough time to prepare meals. However, the amount of time they spend on driving to get the ordered food from outside is almost the same amount of time it takes to cook homemade food. Boiling pasta takes 10–12 minutes and they can utilize the same time to make a salad. Soup is always a good idea; try adding frozen spinach to it, plus an extra can of water and a can of red kidney beans to make a delicious dinner.

The scientist also thinks that children should develop a habit of eating and sleeping on time to prevent obesity. Spending several hours watching TV or at a computer is not healthy. Children need to be engaged in alternative activities. Another option is to have a pet that children can play with and take care of outside.

There are some effective interventions to reduce obesity. Evidence shows that consumption of sugar beverages and energy-dense food predicts an overweight person. Physical activity and sufficient sleep time are also important. Having TV in the bedroom could be detrimental and may interfere with sleep in children. Parents have to listen to the advice given by doctors and set up a healthy home environment, modeling good eating habits and providing healthy food for the children. They need to be actively engaged in building healthy behaviors for their children.

THEORETICAL FRAMEWORK AND SUGGESTIONS FROM RESEARCH

Childhood obesity statistics from 2007 indicate the stunning fact that almost 60 percent of children in America are obese. The rate of overweight children in the United States of America has increased rapidly and it has tripled in the last thirty years (Childhood obesity statistics, 2007). Children with high BMI often become obese adults.

It has been established that nutritious meals are important in the overall development of children. Maslow's (1943) hierarchy of needs stresses the need or desire of academic achievement will not drive a person's thoughts and behaviors until the basic needs are met (Woodhouse & Lamport, 2012). Further, nutrition and academic performance are affected by sociocultural factors. Vygotsky's (1978) sociocultural theories support a person's eating habits. Maslow and Vygotsky provide theoretical perspectives on how food affects students' academic performances. Overall diet quality and academic performance has been studied, and increased fruit and vegetable intake along with reduced dietary fat consumption have been significantly linked to improved academic performance (Florence, Asbridge, and Veugelets, 2008). Moreover, there is direct and negative correlation between fast food consumption and academic performance.

Since children spend a large amount of their waking hours in school, and may consume up to two meals (plus a snack) while at school, researchers and policy makers have begun to look closely at school nutrition policy as an important subject for intervention (Laitsch, 2009). Research has found a correlation between nutrition and students' academic achievements but this relationship is highly underresearched.

According to Sharma et al (2011), good nutrition is vital if one is to travel the road to good health. Further, not only is good nutrition vital for the normal growth of children but it helps to maintain physical and mental fitness throughout their life span.

In one research study, the author and the researcher collected data from forty grade school children enrolled in a summer program. In this public elementary school in New York, where obesity is not an issue, children reported eating healthy food 90 percent of the time. The remaining 10 percent reported that they would occasionally turn to unhealthy foods. They mentioned that they eat outside restaurant food anywhere from zero to three days a week. About 45 percent reported that they are involved in sports or dance activities. The most popular sports were volleyball, basketball, tennis, baseball, football, and soccer. Further, they reported that 100 percent of the children get anywhere from 8–11 hours of sleep daily.

Although the effects of nutrition on health and school performance are often cited, few research studies have examined the effect of nutritious food on students' academic achievement. Another study examined students' overall diet quality, whether it is nutritious or not, and the effect on their academic achievement. Thirty-four third graders who belong to a public Title I school in Queens, New York, participated in this study. Twenty of those participants were from a gifted and talented class and the rest were from a regular third grade class.

The purpose of this study was to examine students' nutritional intake and the effect it had on their academic achievement. The researcher hypothesized that if students eat a healthy and nutritious meal, then they will be in good academic standing. The author asked the question: "Are students who eat more nutritious meals better achievers than students who eat less nutritious meals?"

A meal questionnaire was given to the students which examined what they ate and drank for breakfast, lunch, and dinner. They were also asked whether they liked to eat breakfast, how often they ate fast food, and what their favorite food was. Further, the author observed students in the cafeteria while they were eating lunch to see what they ate and what their attitudes toward the meal were. Moreover, informal interviews were conducted by the researcher with two parents chosen at random, with two randomly selected lunch ladies, and with the gifted students' teacher.

The results indicated that students eating a nutritious diet have a good academic standing. Evidence showed that the gifted class liked to eat breakfast more often than the regular class. Other significant results of this study were that students from the regular class ate more fast food than students from the gifted class; students from the gifted class ate more nutritious foods at dinnertime than students in the regular class. In conclusion, this study indicated the need for the schools to play a major part in educating their students about nutrition so that they can make healthy food choices wherever they are.

Table 2.2. Percentage of Gifted Students Versus Regular Students Who Like to Eat Breakfast

Responses	Gifted	Regular
Almost Never/Sometimes	5%	29%
Almost Always/Often	95%	71%

FREQUENCY OF EATING BREAKFAST

The frequency of eating breakfast was explored in question 1 of the meal questionnaire: Do you like eating breakfast? Breakfast is the most important meal of the day and it fuels the brain and helps to keep students calm so that they can be focused throughout the day. Table 2.2 shows a comparison of the percentage of gifted students and regular students who like to eat breakfast.

The researcher concluded that a significant amount, 95 percent, of students from the gifted class like to eat breakfast, while only 71 percent of the students from the regular class like to eat breakfast.

QUALITY OF BREAKFAST

The author found that cereal, waffles, eggs, and milk were popular breakfast foods. These foods are high in carbohydrates and protein so they were considered nutritious. Table 2.3 shows the percentage of gifted and regular students who ate a nutritious or less nutritious breakfast.

From the result of the data in table 2.3, the researcher concluded that a significant amount, 85 percent, of gifted students versus 57 percent of regular students ate a nutritious breakfast.

The researcher interviewed two of the lunch ladies from the participants' school. The lunch ladies were asked about their feelings about nutrition and student learning. They both emphatically said that it goes hand in hand. They felt that it was important for

Table 2.4. Percentage of Gifted Students Versus Regular Students Who Ate a Nutritious or Less Nutritious Breakfast

Quality of Breakfast	Gifted	Regular
Nutritious (1)	85%	57%
Less Nutritious (2)	15%	43%

students to eat breakfast and, most importantly, a nutritious breakfast which contained fruits and whole grains.

They went on to say that the school serves breakfast to eligible students so they have access to a nutritious breakfast if they participate in the program. One said that at her former school, students would sometimes have chips and soda for breakfast and even they were more alert than those students with empty stomachs.

STUDENTS TAKING SCHOOL LUNCH OR BRINGING LUNCH FROM HOME

Table 2.4 shows that 70 percent of the students from the gifted class participated in the school lunch program while a more significant amount—93 percent—of the regular students participated.

Table 2.3. Percentage of Gifted Students Versus Regular Students Who Take School Lunch or Bring Lunch from Home

Responses	Gifted	Regular
Bring Lunch	30%	7%
Take School Lunch	70%	93%

QUALITY OF LUNCH

Table 2.5 shows the percentage of gifted and regular students who ate a nutritious or less nutritious lunch.

Peanut butter and jelly sandwiches, chicken, rice, dumplings, broccoli, mozzarella sticks, bananas, milk, etc., were foods that students (regular and gifted) all mentioned in the meal questionnaire as typical of what they ate for lunch. The researcher compared students' responses on the questionnaire with the USDA MyPlate food guide recommendations and found that all of the students (100 percent) from the gifted class were consuming nutritious food.

Also the researcher noted what the gifted students wrote that they ate for lunch and whether they participated in the school lunch program or brought lunch from home. The researcher found that either way, the majority of them ate a nutritious lunch. In the case of the regular students, table 2.5 indicates that 86 percent of the students ate a nutritious lunch.

Table 2.5. Percentage of Gifted Students Versus Regular Students Who Ate a Nutritious or Less Nutritious Lunch

Quality of Lunch	Gifted	Regular
Nutritious	100%	86%
Less Nutritious	0%	14%

ADDITIONAL COMMENTARY

The two lunch ladies interviewed were asked whether they think the school provides a nutritious lunch for students. They both affirmed that they did. They said that the school lunch is made up of only whole grains and they try in every way to make the vegetables enticing for the students to eat. They went on to say that they themselves eat school lunch all the time and they feel that it is edible, tasty, and nutritious for the students. A parent with children from the same grade level, chosen at random and interviewed by the researcher, said that her children ate school lunch but that she felt that it could be made more nutritious by adding more fruits and vegetables.

The researcher also observed the thirty-four participants during lunchtime. The researcher noticed that students who brought lunch from home, in comparison to students taking school lunch, had more time to eat most of their lunch before it was time to go out for recess. The researcher asked the lunch ladies whether the students had enough time to eat lunch. They both said that even if they had more time they would still eat the same amount of food because they like to use their time to chat with their classmates.

The researcher also observed that students ate more of the foods they liked (for example, mozzarella sticks) and just took a bite of the foods they didn't really like (for example, broccoli) and threw the rest of their lunch in the trash. Also the researcher observed that students poured out most of the milk they claimed that they drank for lunch. This makes the researcher wonder: how much of the nutritious lunch that students have access to is actually eaten?

The gifted class teacher indicated that she was in agreement with the researcher because she said that although students have access to fruit, vegetables, and whole grains in the cafeteria, it does not mean that they actually eat those foods.

From the interview with the lunch ladies, the researcher found that they believe the school serves a nutritious lunch to its students, which is confirmed by what the students wrote as the foods they consume for lunch. The lunch ladies said every so often they have promotions to help their students make healthy food choices. For example, they have what they called "burger mania" to promote both beef and vegetable burgers. These burgers are considered nutritious because they are served on a whole-wheat bun. The researcher asked the lunch ladies whether students like to eat the vegetable burgers and they said rarely.

One of the lunch ladies went on to say that she usually tries her best to encourage students to eat the food being served for lunch, but that she is afraid that students will go home and tell their parents that the lunch lady is forcing them to eat. When asked if the school sends any information home to parents on nutrition, they said that was not a practice at this school. The gifted class teacher, when asked the same question, said that she does not think the school educates the children specifically on nutrition.

She went on to say, "It is my personal opinion that a PTA meeting should be dedicated towards holding a nutrition workshop for the parents. Kids eat what they are offered by their parents generally speaking and I think the responsibility should fall on them."

The gifted class teacher claimed that during snack time most of her students ate nutritiously, but nevertheless the few who happen to be struggling in school ate foods such as Doritos and Oreos, which are not nutritious. She said she thinks it has mostly to do with a child's parents' style. She also said parents who are on top of everything at school are usually on top of everything about nutrition, too.

The researcher checked math scores attained from the teachers for the gifted and regular students against whether they ate nutritiously or less nutritiously at lunch. When students eat less nutritious food, their achievement decreases. Also the math scores for both gifted and regular students were combined into one large sample and correlation indicates that there is a clear relationship between type of food intake and academic achievement. Just as in the regular students' results, as students eat less nutritious food, their achievement decreases.

There was a significant difference between the fast-food eating habits of gifted (M = 1.8, SD = 0.6) and regular students (M = 3, SD = 1.07), t (32) = –4.04, p < .05. The gifted students in that school ate fast food at a rate of a little less than once a week, while regular students ate it at a rate of a little less than twice a week.

FAVORITE FOOD

The question was "what is your favorite food?" The researcher found that students wrote more than one response to this question but the food that popped up almost all the time for the regular class was pizza. Over 65 percent of the students chose pizza as their favorite food. Pizza can be considered nutritious depending on how it is made but, in the case of these students, their pizza was either from the school lunch or from places like Pizza Hut so their choice of favorite food was not the most nutritious. This clearly sends a message that students need more instruction with regard to nutrition so that they can make healthy food choices.

In the case of the students from the gifted class, 30 percent of the students said pizza was their favorite food. Some of the students from this class made healthy choices, for example, dumplings, curry, and chicken. Although this is a smaller percentage than the students in the general education class, it does not dismiss the need for students to be educated nutritionally so that they can make healthy food choices.

QUALITY OF DINNER

It was found that about 85 percent of the gifted students usually ate a nutritious dinner, while on the other hand, about 50 percent of the regular students did so. This result clearly indicates that parents need to feed their children more nutritiously and help them to make healthy food choices. This is also where school intervention plays an important part. If schools have effective nutrition programs, then students can take that knowledge home and, together with their parents, they can make healthy food choices that will benefit them in the future.

DISCUSSION FROM THE ABOVE RESEARCH

Students in the gifted class had to be high achievers in order to earn a place in that class. The results from the study support the hypothesis that if students eat healthy and nutritious meals, they will, in all probability, be in good academic standing. Shephard (1997) agrees that students who have taken part in a breakfast or physical activity program are calmer in class and more energetic when studying. Thus it is important for students to eat a nutritious breakfast.

The results showed that 95 percent of the students in the gifted class like to eat breakfast versus only 71 percent of the regular class. Students in the gifted class are high achievers and eating a nutritious breakfast obviously helps them to maintain their academic status.

Additionally, this study shows that regular students eat fast food more frequently than the gifted students. This finding indicates the need for schools to educate their students nutritionally so that they can make healthy food choices and perform better academically.

Iron is vital for proper brain function. Also iodine deficiencies in the early childhood years have similarly been associated with difficulty in cognition and school achievement. Adequate daily supply of proteins, complex carbohydrates, and calcium is considered essential for students' academic success (livestrong.com, 2011).

According to the lunch ladies who were interviewed, schools are trying their best to encourage students to eat healthy foods. Students taking school breakfast and lunch have access to food containing whole grain and less sugar. Ninety-three percent of the students from the regular class versus 70 percent from the gifted class take school lunch. Thus, whether students are from the gifted or the regular class, results indicate that they have access to nutritious lunch.

Nevertheless, the researcher found from observation in the school's cafeteria that students tend to only eat what they like and just take a bite of what they don't like and dump the rest in the trash. Also the gifted class teacher said in her interview that even though students may have access to fruit and vegetables, it does not mean that they actually consume them.

Eating nutritiously is of great importance because it has a direct impact on academic achievement and can affect students' school performance. According to Sharma et al. (2011), good nutrition is vital if one is to travel the road to good health. Therefore, good nutrition helps to maintain the physical and mental fitness in adults throughout their life span.

Michelle Obama (2011) reinforced that "We can all agree that in the wealthiest nation on Earth, all children should have the basic nutrition they need to learn and grow and to pursue their dreams, because in the end, nothing is more important than the health and well-being of our children. . . . These are the basic values that we all share, regardless of race, party, religion. This is what we share" (Fitness Quotes by Michelle Obama, March 23, 2011).

Thus, in order to produce great achievers, schools have the opportunity together with parents to educate their students/children nutritionally so that they can make healthy food choices.

A NEW GAME PLAN

Creating a supportive school and family environment can help children develop healthy habits and learn how to live a healthy lifestyle. Teachers can provide information to parents on childhood obesity and prevention, as well as resources to make parents aware of lifestyle practices they can implement in their family so children learn to make healthier choices in their diet and engage in physical activities.

Healthy habits can be implemented across curricula in classrooms to extend children's knowledge of nutrition and physical activity. Nutrition can be incorporated into the classroom on a daily basis by having lunch and/or snack set up in different food groups. Physical activity can be included in the schedule for each day, and during this time teachers can instruct students on simple exercises they can do in the classroom and also at home to promote movement.

In a unit on nutrition, literacy can be incorporated by having students develop their own personal health goals, and then creating graphic organizers to plan to meet their goals. Nutrition instruction can be incorporated into math by having students examine nutritional values of various foods and drinks and discuss how the values can help identify what healthier choices are.

Science can be included in nutrition instruction through conducting experiments that break down components of food so students can observe how unhealthy foods and drinks metabolize in our bodies. Social studies can be included in nutrition instruction extended outside the classroom. Students can research health resources and organic farms within the community that may be useful to them, and then the classes can take community walks to visit the places and find out more information about new initiatives in growing organic foods.

There are a variety of ways teachers can integrate nutrition education in the classroom. It can be incorporated in math, science, English language arts, and many other activities.

Math

There are many activities and lessons that can be taught in the nutrition topic. Sorting real fruits and vegetables by color and/or shape, or sorting pictures of all the food groups as a receptive activity can be instructional for younger children. For older children, naming the food in the food group and creating a chart of similarities and differences of different kinds of fruits and vegetables is a good activity.

In an apples lesson or unit, different types of apples can be examined as well as the parts of the apple, where each apple comes from, etc. Students can also have a tasting party and complete a class bar graph of their favorite types of apples. You can also make applesauce or an apple pie, and the children can learn about measurements for cooking.

Science

Children can grow a vegetable, like a green bean plant, that they can personally take care of. The classroom can have different herbs or flowering plants on the window sill where sunlight comes in. Lessons can be taught about fruits, vegetables, and the human body. These units can teach a variety of science topics.

Water Station

If a water station is allowed in the classroom, it can be used to practice pouring water into different containers. A lesson on how important water is for your body and health can be taught. We can teach how to substitute sugary drinks and soda for water. We can also integrate literacy and learn new words such as hydrate, dehydrate, and quench.

RAISING PARENT AWARENESS ABOUT THE IMPORTANCE OF CHILDREN'S NUTRITION

There are many ways to incorporate nutrition decisions in everyday life. Make the child's learning about healthy things in the house fun. Teach your child to help cook with you or to help you make a salad, a fruit salad, or pumpkin soup. Parents and teachers can also teach children about how different fruits and vegetables look, or use all five senses to describe the fruits and vegetables and how they are good for you. You can also make your own cookbook.

Using a well-developed method of teaching parents and adding health and physical education to curriculum will help children develop healthy habits. One such program is the Healthy Children, Healthy Families: Parents Making A Difference! (HCHF), a well-thought-out plan to educate those who can most affect change. Particularly designed for low-income families, it is a parent education curriculum taught in a series of workshops that have been developed to address six key nutritional and physical activity behavioral objectives along with parenting strategies. The results of these workshops show an improvement in overall health of children in the participating families (Lent, Hill, Dollahite, Wolfe, & Dickin, 2012).

Another program designed to help provide nutrition education to children is the Newtown Kids' Programme (NKP). Through the school nurse and health professional referrals, NKP was developed to help educate children and parents about best practices for a healthy lifestyle.

Physical activity sessions are scheduled after school and on weekends to accommodate families. The sessions include fun, team-based physical activities for children in schools and other community centers. There are also educational sessions designed for children and parents as well that focus on healthy eating habits. This program saw a rise in self-esteem amongst participating children, and an increase in positive attitudes toward physical activity. The main goal of NKP is to help children increase their desire for and understanding of physical activity and healthy habits (Fraser, Lewis, & Manby, 2012).

Federal and state laws are a more permanent approach to making an impact on fighting obesity. Mandates on school food along with the elimination of physical education in some schools should not be tolerated. Communities need to put pressure on district leaders to bring about positive change in schools regarding higher standards of healthy nutrition and physical activity. Following are some of the initiatives taken:

• A pilot program called CATCH (Coordinated Approach To Child Health for Early Childhood) has been implemented in preschool to create a nutrition and physical activity curriculum. CATCH is developed into four groupings: classroom curriculum, physical activity, parent education, and teacher training. The bulk of the material includes educational stan-

dards that are required in preschool using nutritional information as a tool to educate young children. All subject matter can
be implemented into the topic of nutrition (Sharma, Chuang,
& Hedberg, 2011).

- The National Heart Savers Association of Omaha, Nebraska,
  has implemented a health curriculum for kindergarten through
  eighth grade to help teachers integrate health and nutrition
  into the classroom lessons. They have laid out an in-depth
  grade-by-grade breakdown of different activities to incorporate into academic learning which emphasize the importance
  of good nutrition and physical education. Activities include a
  word scramble with fruits as the words or taking one's pulse
  to learn mathematics. Any subject matter can incorporate nutrition at any grade level.

Educators and parents can help children develop healthy habits by
teaching them about the food groups. They can also show and
explain to children what healthy foods (fish, vegetables, fruits,
grains, milk, cheese, etc.) are as opposed to those we should not be
frequently eating (potato chips, soda, juice, candy, chocolate, etc.)
Interactive classroom play can help children better understand the
concept of healthy food versus unhealthy food.

Educators can make a big difference. Teaching students about
good nutrition is critical to helping them make healthy food
choices. The challenge is for classroom teachers to incorporate nutrition lessons into a school day. A teacher can connect healthy
eating into core subjects like science and social studies. When students bring unique foods from home in their lunches, the teacher
can create a mini "food study" around it. A teacher can talk about
or show food by season. Students can categorize food by color,
such as red pepper or strawberry for red.

In one instance on Halloween, the teacher and her class studied
orange and black foods that come from the earth; on Valentine's
Day, students could learn about pink and red foods. Occasionally,

the class could look at the sticker on a piece of fruit to find out where it comes from, point the area out on the classroom globe and discuss where the food normally grows, explaining why that type of fruit only grows in certain areas and climates.

Nutrition builds strong bones and provides the proper nutrients that the human body needs. All children have unique nutritional requirements. Teaching children about nutrition when they are young is essential for their future. The younger they learn about a healthy lifestyle, the happier and healthier they will be!

TEACHERS TAKING AN ACTIVE ROLE

Teachers should take the extra step to incorporate nutritional lessons and activities on a weekly basis. Educating children about nutrition will make a difference in students' health and in their lives. There are so many fun-filled activities that students can participate in while learning about a healthy lifestyle. While teaching a nutrition unit, a teacher discussed with her students certain emotions that come with being healthy and listening to their responses was wonderful!

Some of the responses from the children were "I feel happy when I exercise!" "Drinking water makes me feel good!" "Mommy and Daddy are very happy when I eat my vegetables at dinner!" After such a discussion, the teacher could review the five food groups, going around the room so that students can talk as a class about each group.

It is a good idea to write a letter home to inform the parents that this week is going to be called "nutrition week." Instead of juice for their child's beverage, ask parents to send water and healthy snacks.

One teacher narrated the following that she did with her students:

The activity was called "Find the Apple." The teacher went outside to the playground with the children. Prior to going out to the playground, the teacher and her assistants hid the apples around the playground. The students had to walk, hop, and crawl looking for these apples. The teacher rang a bell each time that they had to switch up their physical movement (walk, hop, or crawl). This kept the children interested in the game and eager to find the apples. They also did this game with other fruits and vegetables to teach children about healthy food. This activity was followed by reading a book: *Apples* by Gail Gibbons.

Another activity is to raise awareness among students that food can be grown and it does not come out of a can or from the grocery store. So it is important to grow a vegetable garden at home or in the school yard. Many children believe that milk comes out of a carton kept in the refrigerator. Children should get the exposure to go to the farm and see how we get milk from the cows.

The next activity that the teacher did with the students was to promote physical activity by cutting out a bubble wrap in the shape of a fruit. The students reviewed the different shapes of fruits and then began the game. The teacher played music for the children and they were able to walk, jump, hop, or dance across the bubble wrap. When the music stopped, they told the teacher what shape they were on and what fruit it represented. They loved hearing the popping sounds that the bubble wrap made. The children loved dance time.

On the last day of nutrition week, the teachers did two activities to really end the week off right. They played a game called "healthy eating hopscotch." This game promoted healthy eating and also enhanced balance and strength for the young children. The teacher drew 10 connected boxes with duct tape on the carpet. She then demonstrated the activity by throwing a bean bag with a picture of a fruit or vegetable on it, landing it on one of the boxes. The students hopped through the boxes and then turned back to the beginning while picking up the healthy bean bag.

The last game was "the missing fruit game." This game was similar to the first game that they played but it included "fruit game cards." The teacher first hid plastic fruit around the classroom. They then talked about the different fruit game cards and how important each fruit is to our bodies. To begin the game, the teacher held up a fruit game card. If the fruit game card was a banana, they had to find the banana hidden in the classroom by marching, hopping, skipping, or crawling.

There are different ways educators and parents can help children to develop healthy habits. Both parents and teachers should be role models for their children. Children love to imitate adults. Keeping healthy snacks in your house or classroom is one way of showing children what they should be eating. Making meals a part of a child's daily routine will also help them make healthier choices.

Teachers can provide workshops for parents, as well as students, to discuss healthy eating habits. Educators can provide families with the MyPlate food diagram and explain what types and how much of different foods from each food group they should be consuming on a daily basis. They should discuss what a balanced meal looks like for breakfast, lunch, and dinner. Combinations of protein, fruit, vegetables, and carbohydrates can also be suggested in a meal plan format to give parents a starting point at home.

Teachers can provide lists of healthy snacks that can be sent into homes. Once the parents are made aware of the healthy food, they can incorporate healthy snacks into the daily routines with their children. Once these healthy decisions are made for a child, they will learn to make the same decisions when they have a choice. Katz et al. (2011) conducted a study to evaluate the effects of a nutrition education program designed to teach elementary school students and their parents, and to distinguish between more healthy and less healthy choices in diverse food categories.

Katz et al. (2011) suggests that programs should directly cultivate practical and "actionable" skills related to daily physical activity, healthful eating, or both. In addition, programs should reach both students and their parents so that families may reinforce what is taught in school in the home environment.

New York City public schools offer a wide range of wellness programs. The Department of Education (DOE) Wellness Programs, such as Move-to-Improve, the School Wellness Council Grant Program, and the Health Education Leadership Program, are part of a larger commitment to raising student achievement levels and combating the childhood obesity epidemic.

Comprehensive health education begins in elementary school and continues through high school. It includes age-appropriate lessons on injury prevention, mental and emotional health, nutrition, tobacco, alcohol and other drugs, family health and sexuality, HIV/AIDS, and personal and consumer health.

Mandatory HIV/AIDS lessons for kindergarten through twelfth grade are supported by a curriculum that offers age-appropriate lessons. Fitness and physical education programs focus on a health-related fitness education curriculum. Integration of NYC FITNESSGRAM is a standardized fitness assessment tool drawn from decades of research and designed specifically for New York City public school students. The CHAMPS Middle School Sports and Fitness Program also has physical activity programs for adolescents.

According to the Center for Collaborative Solutions (CCS), "students tend to benefit the most when they are involved in projects or activities that last long enough for them to acquire new knowledge, develop and strengthen their skills, become excited about learning and experience a sense of being able to carry something through to completion." Teachers can integrate fun and innovative activities that include a variety of subjects. For example, children can learn to count vegetables, they can play games that include matching and sorting food items, they can create patterns with food items.

Cooking or creating snacks with children can develop their math skills and help them to learn how to follow directions. It also assists and improves their social skills because students can talk amongst themselves and teachers can ask many questions while cooking or creating the snack. For example, teachers and students can make a banana boat together where the children slice bananas in half and then lengthwise and add apple pieces for a mast, or they can make a fruit salad or their own MyPlates.

Teachers can take students to the grocery store and identify healthy food items. Teachers can have a pretend grocery store activity in their classrooms with designated responsibilities for each student within the store; this activity would help students improve their math skills.

Students can conduct science experiments such as planting a bean seed or assisting with a gardening project (with parent's consent). Children's books on nutrition can also be read to reinforce and strengthen children's language arts, math, science, social studies, and comprehension skills simultaneously. Nature walks and trips to educational museums or facilities engage and retain children's attention; they will be eager to learn, thus making their experience more enjoyable.

This notion is supported in the Center for Collaborative Solutions guidebook which mentions the following: "Offering a wide variety of opportunities for children and young people in your program to engage in hands-on, experiential learning that allows them to build, master, and internalize new concepts and skills, and share ideas and experiences with their peers keeps them interested and growing. When activities are age appropriate and engaging, students will be much more attentive, receptive, and excited about learning, and they'll learn more."

Teachers can work to develop a unit plan on nutrition (see appendix B) which focuses on the five food groups while incorporating proper exercise and movement activities as well as proper hygiene tips, all while integrating math, science, English, and social studies.

This unit plan on nutrition will teach students the importance of eating protein, vegetables, fruits, grains, and dairy products. It will help students understand why each of these food groups helps their bodies function properly.

Teachers can provide students with all of this information by planning a unit on "The Importance of Being Healthy." The unit will consist of five lessons and each day a food group will be introduced. In order to provide nutrition education for parents and their children, teachers can offer "nutrition bags" to be sent home with students. Parents will be given the proper resources to learn how to implement healthy eating habits at home with their children.

Inside the nutrition bags will be fun activities for students and parents to do together, including movement activities, recipes, and educational tools for each food group. Parents will have an evaluation sheet to fill out which will help the teacher and parents communicate what the children learned. The nutrition bag is a great tool in helping teachers and families unite to provide a healthy lifestyle for children and to promote "The Importance of Being Healthy."

Teachers can teach a unit on nutrition via spelling or by reading stories that talk about nutrition and healthy food. Further, there are scenarios as to how families can teach their children about healthy

Table 2.6. Food Groups and Benefits

Proteins	Grains	Vegetables and Fruits	Dairy Products
Help build, maintain, and heal muscles. Examples include meats, fish, nuts, seeds, milk, beans, and cheese.	Help give you energy. Examples include cereals and grains.	Help reduce risk of heart disease, including stroke and heart attack, as well as protect against certain types of cancer.	Help improve bone health and may reduce risk of osteoporosis.

eating. The following are samples of nutrition lesson plans that span the subjects of English, math, science, and social studies.

For example, in English class, students can read articles about nutrition, then discuss and write poems about what was learned. For math, have an "unbake" sale where you sell fruit or fruit kebabs and veggie garden cups. For science, advocate for a greenhouse and plant veggies—usually tomatoes and cucumbers are easy to grow. With science, children can be shown or conduct their own experiments with different foods, or they can learn about the effects/possible harm that certain foods have on their bodies. Through the science section, we can also discuss obesity, type 2 diabetes, or other health issues that arise from long-term consumption of unhealthy foods.

For social studies, discuss with students the main healthy crops that grow in a particular region. Further, teachers can take a class trip to a farmers' market. Teachers can integrate the unit of nutrition across curricula through lesson plans centered on the five food groups. With social studies, we can discuss how certain foods are grown and harvested in different parts of the world. Different fruits and vegetables can be examined, including some that can only be grown in certain climates, such as tropical fruit.

There are many ways that parents can encourage their kids to eat healthy foods. Parents can take their children grocery shopping and let them pick out healthy food. Parents can also encourage kids to garden or take them to local farms so they can see where vegetables and fruits come from. Parents should always have healthy snacks available at home (as opposed to unhealthy snacks) and teachers should give students the option to choose what snack they would like to eat.

Parents can make smoothies or freshly squeezed fruit juices to offer their children if they do not like eating fruits and vegetables so that they still get the nutrients they need. Natural or organic foods should be offered to young children because they do not contain harmful pesticides. Teachers can help provide nutrition education to children by discussing healthy eating habits and encouraging parents to bring in only healthy food for their child to eat while in school.

One activity that adults can do with children is to fill up a lunchbox with healthy foods and drinks, also making a chart with five days' worth of healthy choices. Another activity is for children to pretend to get ready for a vacation and pack nonperishable food items, games, and sports equipment or dance items, planning and creating a ten-day chart of foods and activities for the imagined trip.

DISCUSSION QUESTIONS

1. What are some of the experts' comments on preventing obesity among young children?
2. How would you promote health and nutrition education among young children to prevent obesity?
3. With nutrition as a unit, how can teachers teach across curricula (English, math, science, and social studies)?

REFERENCES

Florence, M. D., M. Asbridge, and P. J. Veugelers. 2008. Diet quality and academic performance. *Journal of School Health* 78 (4).

Fraser, C., K. Lewis, and M. Manby. 2012. Steps in the right direction, against the odds, an evaluation of a community-based programme aiming to reduce inactivity and improve health and morale in overweight and obese school-aged children. *Children & Society* (August). National Children's Bureau and Blackwell Publishing Limited.

Katz, D. L., C. S. Katz, J. A. Treu, J. Reynolds, V. Njike, J. Walker, E. Smith, and J. Michael. 2011. Teaching healthful food choices to elementary school students and their parents: The nutrition detectives™ program. *Journal of School Health* 81 (1): 21–28.

Laitsch, D. 2009. Nutrition and schools' knowledge summary/Nutrition et sommaire des connaissance scolaires. *McGill Journal of Education* (online) 44 (2) (Spring): 261–85.

Lent, M., T. F. Hill, J. S. Dollahite, W. S. Wolfe, and K. L. Dickin. 2012. Healthy children, healthy families: Parents making a difference! A curriculum integrating key nutrition, physical activity, and parenting practices to help prevent childhood obesity. *Journal of Nutrition Education and Behavior* 44 (1) (January–February): 90–2. doi: 10.1016/j.jneb.2011.02.011. Epub 2011 Sep 6.

Maslow, A. 1943. A theory of human motivation. *Psychological Review* (50): 370–96. Retrieved from http://psychclassics.yorku.ca/Maslow/motivation.htm.

Sharma, S., R. Chuang, and A. M. Hedberg. 2011. Pilot-testing CATCH early childhood: A preschool-based healthy nutrition and physical activity program. *American Journal of Health Education* 42 (1): 12–23.

Shephard, R. J. 1997. Curricular physical activity and academic performance. *Pediatric Exercise Science* 9: 113–26.

Woodhouse, A., and M. A. Lamport. 2012. The relationship of food and academic performance: A preliminary examination of the factors of nutritional neuroscience, malnutrition and diet adequacy. *Christian Perspectives in Education: Send out your light and your truth! Let them guide me, Psalm: 43:3*, 5(1): 1–15.

Vygotsky, L. S. 1978. *Mind in Society.* Cambridge, MA: Harvard University Press.

Yadav, M. P., D. Johnston, A. T. Hotchkiss, and K. B. Hicks. 2005. Corn fiber gum: A potential gum arabic replacer for beverage flavor emulsification. Agricultural Research Service, US Department of Agriculture.

WEBSITES

http://www.livestrong.com/article/389438-research-on-nutrition-school-performance/

http://www.fitnessquotes.org/fitness-quotes-by-michelle-obama/

3

IMPORTANCE OF PHYSICAL EXERCISE

LEARNING OBJECTIVES

1. Importance of physical exercise for young children.
2. How can sports, yoga, music, and dance contribute to the aspect of physical exercise among children?

The World Health Organization (WHO) states that physical activity for children, particularly sports play, is crucial in the fight against the rise in obesity worldwide. Sports and other physical activities contribute to our social and mental health. Physical exercise plays a key feature in the overall well-being of a human being. The recommended amount of physical activity a child should engage in is one to two hours of active play each day.

Conklin, Marshak, and Meyer (2004) suggest ways to incorporate healthy nutrition among children. "Vending machines should be stocked with healthy fruit snacks and beverages, trail mixes, dried fruit, 100% fruit juices, baked chips, etc. Classroom and physical education teachers, food service managers, and other staff should work together to ensure the flow of nutrition throughout the curriculum."

According to Massey-Stokes (2002), "Good health is essential for effective learning, by eating well, and engaging in other healthy

behaviors, children can boost their performance level and successfully master key growth development tasks. Undernutrition can be
present in both 'malnourished' youth who do not have enough to
eat, [and in others who] . . . consume nutrient-deficient diets." The
author further mentions that nutrition is important because children
need sufficient nutrients in their bodies, especially iron. Iron deficiency causes students to feel fatigued, reduces their attention span,
and decreases their work capacity.

Massey-Stokes (2002) also states that proper nutrition can help
to decrease children's risk for four of the nation's diet-related
chronic diseases: coronary heart disease, specific cancers, strokes,
and type 2 diabetes. Further, Fisher and Madeson (2007) suggest
that "both friend, and family support are significantly correlated
with physical activity among youth."

Today, less than half of youth aged 6 to 17 years meet these
recommendations (Dalton, 2013). The alternative—ongoing, sedentary behavior—leads to negative effects on physical and mental
health. Not only does physical activity build strong bones and reduce risk factors for obesity and chronic disease, engagement in
regular physical exercise helps improve concentration, memory,
and classroom behavior.

Some may argue that physical education in school takes away
from academics. This argument is based on the idea that the less
time devoted to rigorous academics, the less a child will learn.

Research has suggested otherwise. Abadie and Brown (2010)
note that, "When a physical education class is incorporated into the
academic curriculum, there is not a reduction in academic performance in traditional academic programs though class time devoted
to traditional academics is reduced because of the introduction of
the physical education class . . . physical activity also has been
demonstrated to promote mental functioning central to cognitive
development."

Children who spend less time exercising performed worse on test scores in both math and reading compared to their more active peers. A study published by the Public Library of Science found a positive relationship between aerobic fitness, learning, and memory in a group of fourth grade students, indicating reduction in physical education in schools may hinder academic performance for developing children. Therefore, schools should not only provide physical education but also promote exercise for academic success. In response to this need, federally funded programs, such as Let's Move! Active Schools, and the Presidential Youth Fitness Program, have been incorporated in schools across the country.

In school, recess is an important activity for healthy childhood. Many schools have decreased, if not eliminated recess. Recess allows student to develop physically and socially in ways they cannot elsewhere. The playground area should also be an interactive area for children to engage in physical activity.

Despite federally funded programs in schools to promote physical activity, schools may face limitations in this area and consequentially are unable to provide children with the recommended amount of physical exercise per day.

At home, children can be encouraged to exercise by incorporating physical activity into the whole family's lifestyle. Family outings, bike rides, walks, and various active play times are small ways to get kids moving. Other strategies for parents include limiting TV and computer time, choosing the right activities for a child's age, and giving kids plenty of time to be active while keeping the focus on the fun.

Communities need to be included in the promotion of physical activity for children because many opportunities exist outside home and school. Community activity programs can help children improve their physical well-being, developing social skills in the process. When collaborating with schools, communities can work toward motivating children to engage in extracurricular activities that take place in a safe environment.

Schools can educate children on the need for physical activity while providing them with information on community activity programs which complement the instruction given at school. This allows the community to establish relationships with schools and parents in which children are accounted for in all areas of life. This can be done by a team of volunteers organizing and planning various informational sessions about the available physical activity clubs, teams, and programs.

Having an established community sports program is a positive step toward promoting a healthy lifestyle; a child's environmental setting can offer many opportunities for exercise. However, activity programs often require special equipment or transportation that may be beyond a family's financial ability.

Communities should ensure that students have access to these programs. By seeking the assistance and donations of other community members, such as business owners, accommodations can be made so that all interested students can participate. Partnerships with local businesses to create low-cost options for such activities benefit all involved. It can also be a way to encourage school, home, and communities to make a difference in their own neighborhoods (Beighle & Johnson, 2012).

The positive effects of sports participation contribute to physical well-being and character development of young children. For instance, a soccer player commented: "Soccer has taught me to be a team player, hard-working, and respectful." The impact of sports on this soccer player's life was fueled by his competitive drive and motivation to succeed.

However, he shared that motivation does not have to come from competition; rather, the social aspect can motivate a child to join a team. Then the goal for an individual is to be with peers, and also to enjoy the physical exercise. Getting out to play on a team is a great way for kids to be healthy.

Sustaining consistent physical exercise at school, home, and in the community is vital because it serves as a concrete foundation for a healthy life. Physical exercise promotes healthy growth and development. It helps people achieve and maintain a healthy weight, confidence, and self-esteem. It can also relieve stress and promote relaxation. It can be a detriment to illness and lifelong diseases such as type 2 diabetes and cardiovascular disorders. Physical exercise helps build stronger bones, muscles, core strength, posture, balance, and coordination.

In addition, physical exercise can positively influence our cognitive processes by establishing connections between different parts of our brains, thus increasing our concentration and thinking skills. Individuals who are physically active are likely to develop good social skills as they are more prone to participate in many activities within their community, such as marathons for positive causes or volunteering within the community. New York Cares, for example, has plenty of physical activities within the community to help children and special education children, such as working out with Achilles Kids.

Physical activity is a very important part of life from birth. At home, it ensures that children are staying healthy and developing at an appropriate rate. In school, it is extremely important in terms of social development, as well as instruction during physical education classes. In the community it is a great way to become involved through activities like Little League or Police Athletic League. Aside from personal involvement, a physically active community may make more health-conscious choices when it comes to instituting health-related programs.

Some ways to help children be active are by providing students with the opportunity to join sports, practice yoga or dance at home, and engage in free play at school during gym and recess. Sports, yoga, music, and dance enhance the physical aspect of exercise for children by focusing on their gross and fine motor skills, thus improving their agility and coordination capabilities, while simultaneously fostering development of social skills.

Multiple benefits to having your child join a sports activity include daily exercise, developing a routine and structure, acquiring knowledge on how to strengthen the body and maintain it, learning to make healthy food choices, understanding the importance of working with a team, preparing both mentally and physically for practices and games, and following safety guidelines to prevent injury.

Physical activity in basketball promotes healthy eating in order to maintain high performance and muscle recovery. When students have a proper diet plan, they are able to perform well, remain fit and focused, and be consistent with their meal choices. They are educated on what helps them remain both physically and mentally prepared for practice and games. Participation in sports helps students build and learn exercise routines, maintain flexibility, muscle definition, and burn calories, and become cognizant of the functions and limitations of their bodies.

Sports also provide students with other physical perks such as keeping one's metabolism going on a consistent basis, releasing endorphins, burning calories, and creating a proper rest cycle. Students can exercise by running, shooting baskets, sprinting, pushing, pulling, bending, diving, and hanging as well as many other activities.

Yoga is a very good form of exercise that keeps the body and mind healthy. A way to unite body and mind, yoga also helps children to manage stress through breathing, meditation, and movement. It helps to build concentration, increase confidence, and develop positive self-image. In a school setting, yoga offers a way to exercise in the classroom if the gym is not available. It gives an alternate method of handling challenges in the classroom. Yoga helps children build strength and energizes the body and the mind. Yoga aids in digestion and in maintaining a healthy weight.

Children's overall balance improves, along with their foot-eye and hand-eye coordination, when they exercise regularly. Children's spatial coordination is also enhanced when doing physical exercise. Dance is a great way to keep kids active. It provides students with the opportunity to learn how their bodies move while keeping them in shape.

In her article on dance, Dow (2010) advocates for the implementation of dance throughout the school day: "Keeping children active is a crucial part of addressing this health crisis and the good news is that teachers don't have to find extra time to add dance to the day. You can incorporate it anytime, in a small space, for greetings, circle time, transitions, or waking up from a nap" (Dow, 2010). She describes simple ways to keep kids active throughout the entire school day. Dancing would allow children to be more in touch with rhythm and improve their mood and self-confidence as music usually produces positive feelings within us. Physical exercise also releases endorphins which boost the children's self-esteem and sense of well-being, and improve muscle tone throughout their bodies.

Children with intellectual disabilities have a weaker capacity for physical activity due to issues related to muscle weakness. The difficulty in beginning physical activity may discourage those children from continuing in fitness programs; however, more exercise can actually help improve physical weaknesses over time. Flexibility, resilience, balance, and endurance will increase when children are involved in physical exercise. A well-designed plan must be created with the ability and functionality of each child in mind (Golubovic, Maksimovic, Golubovic, & Glumbic, 2012). It has been found that obesity is prevalent in children who are blind (Guha, 2015).

Physical exercise, sports, or music is very important for all children, but especially for children who are blind or visually impaired, as many of them have overweight or obesity issues. Blind children and adolescents are less physically active than those with low vision (Greguol, Gobbi, & Carraro, 2014).

Physical activity influences the body image of children and adolescents with visual impairment (Greguol, Gobbi, & Carraro, 2014). Some possible sports activities for these children include running, jumping, and playing cricket. Children who are visually impaired can play cricket by listening for a sound; they hear the sound and then know when to strike the bat. Outside, children who are visually impaired can play with a ball that has a bell inside. Children roll the ball on the ground and run in the direction of the ball when they hear it. Weight training is another way to address obesity issues.

With help, children can enjoy planting seeds and then enjoy fruits and vegetables from their gardens. Children at school and at home should get an opportunity to grow fruits or vegetables, either on the playground or in pots inside the classroom.

Children as young as three years of age are increasingly experiencing traumatic events that lead to post-traumatic stress disorder (PTSD), anxiety, and depression. These issues are difficult to overcome and can stay with a child for years. Physical exercise has been shown to reduce the effects of these conditions and in some cases to virtually eliminate them.

By implementing more physical education into the curriculum in schools, in coordination with families involving their children in physical activity, there is evidence that the rate at which children are experiencing PTSD symptoms might be decreased. "The endorphin hypothesis maintains that exercise increases beta-endorphin levels and that these elevations account for improvements" (Motta, McWilliams, Schwartz, & Cavera, 2012).

Sports provide children with many life skills and lead to a healthy lifestyle. Other physical activity that should be incorporated into all early childhood curricula is dance and movement. The creative art form of movement provides young children with many academic as well as physical benefits. Movement incorporates individual style and ability in a way that with any lesson, flexibility can be made to allow all students to participate with an equal level of benefit (Bergstein, 2010).

Children enjoy challenges and respond well to movement activities. Teachers can incorporate movement in their classrooms to benefit classroom management and to keep children focused. Incorporating any physical activity into the school day will benefit the development of the child.

Experts in the field of physical training agree that children who become involved in these activities learn lifelong lessons as to how the body performs. Studies indicate that children involved in physical activity will continue some form of exercise as adults, will have a lower body-fat percentage, and will eat a more balanced diet.

Early childhood services should offer a wide choice of play-based, physically active learning experiences that build on children's interests, abilities, identities, and knowledge. Physical activity in childcare needs to be made up of both structured physical activity and unstructured, spontaneous activity.

Educators can encourage children to participate in physical activity to motivate them to turn away from drugs and alcohol and to lead healthy lifestyles. Sports can make a tremendous contribution to physical exercise and healthy living. One purpose is to teach inner-city kids not only how to have a safe life away from violence and drugs but to educate them in being active and healthy. Sports provide them with techniques on how to execute plans that they can use in their everyday lives.

Physical activity is an important way to prevent childhood obesity. The vast majority of studies indicate that children who participate in sports have a lower body mass index compared to children who do not participate. However, each child is unique and should be treated differently, depending on age, sex, body weight, and other characteristics that may influence their relationship with physical activity.

Exercise is important at home because children follow the example of their parents. Parents should model and encourage exercise by working out with their child, enrolling them in sports programs, and encouraging outdoor play. Parents should encourage their children to find a sport that builds on their talents and is rewarding. Parents need to make it a priority to start engaging in some of these activities with their children.

Riding bikes to the park or through the neighborhood, taking walks or hikes together, climbing stairs instead of using an elevator, swimming, playing, or practicing sports together are all fun and healthy ways to be active as a family.

HAVING FUN WITH SPORTS

For kids, having fun is the biggest key! Stop thinking of it as "exercise" and think of it as playing. Expending energy is what we are after. Daily physical activity significantly helps maintain a healthy weight. Physical activity, however, does not mean only organized sports, but any kind of movement, like walking and playing.

Children can participate in organized sports such as soccer, baseball, or gymnastics, but jumping rope, skipping, relay races, riding bikes, dizzy bat race, obstacle courses, etc., are all considered physical activity.

The best way to make children become active agents of healthy behavior is to show them how much fun physical activity can be. By demonstrating to children that being physically active is not a chore, they are much more likely to develop a love for healthy activities.

When working with children who have health issues, physical education teachers can make sure that the directions to the entire class include instructions such as an optional break if a student feels overwhelmed by the activity. This way, all students can participate at their own level and not feel left out if they need a break.

According to a physical education teacher, children participate more in the class when music is being played. His classes are for children with autism, thus his physical education program is based largely on coordination and gross motor skills. He uses a number of stations that include various activities. For instance, he uses one exercise station as a cardio area, one for upper body coordination or strength, and another for lower body coordination or strength.

Children spend many hours a day in school, and they also have seemingly unlimited amounts of energy. The energy that children have should be released in physical activities such as dance, exercise, and sports. Not only does physical activity in school help keep students fit but it helps them cool down and focus on the next academic task. Physical exercise in schools is a major concern for parents today. NPR/Robert Wood Johnson Foundation/Harvard School of Public Health (HSPH) polled 1,368 parents of public school children in grades K–12 on a range of issues around education and health in their child's school.

One in four parents (25 percent) said their child's school gives too little emphasis to physical education, compared with one in seven who say the same thing about reading and writing (14 percent) or math (15 percent). In addition, about three in ten parents (28 percent) give a low grade (C, D, or F) to their child's school on providing enough time for physical education, while almost seven in ten parents (68 percent) report that their child's school does not provide daily physical education classes (Datz, 2013).

New York City teachers are now being encouraged under state regulations to provide an ample amount of physical activity each day for their students. However, parents should encourage exercise at home as well. Sports, yoga, music, and dance are fun ways a child can exercise and keep active.

Staying at a healthy weight is all about energy balance; energy (or calories) in versus energy (calories) out. Consumption of 3,500 calories equals one pound. The foods and drinks we consume give us energy, but we need to be smart about what we are consuming so we are getting enough carbohydrates, proteins, and fats without consuming extra calories. For example, a 20-ounce bottle of soda contains 250 calories without any nutritional value. Therefore, with every 20-ounce soda consumed in a day, that is 250 empty calories (no nutrient value) added to our total caloric intake.

To maintain current weight, a person must expend as many calories as they bring in during the day; therefore, adults and children need to be physically active every day in order to maintain weight, much less to lose weight. Unfortunately, children are consuming less milk—which contains nutrients, protein, carbohydrates, minimal fat (if 1% or 2% milk), as well as some vitamins and minerals—and more soda throughout the day. Each 12-ounce can of soda consumed on a regular basis has been shown to increase the risk of obesity by 60 percent.

Parents should encourage cardiovascular types of activity as well as strength building exercises since both are vital to overall health. However, the majority of the 60 minutes should be cardiovascular, especially for those trying to control weight. Strength exercises like push-ups or lunges ensure healthy bones and muscles; however, cardiovascular activities are most important for heart health and maintaining a healthy weight.

The exercises should be cardiovascular and should be the kind of activities that children enjoy such as soccer, running, jumping rope, and swimming laps. Again, it has to be fun or they won't want to do it. The instructor has to be creative and make games out of the activities. Often overweight children don't want to play sports or participate in games because they are afraid they will be ridiculed by other children. Therefore, it is important to do things to make overweight children more apt to participate in games or sports. A variety of things can be done to help overweight children build confidence and have fun.

One way is to change the rules of typical games so everyone is starting off on the same playing field. For example, when playing baseball, make everyone bat with their weakest hand and then run backwards to the bases. This makes the game more fun and less about who is the most talented. Another idea to initially engage children and make them feel successful is to have them play some of the active games on Wii, such as boxing or Wii Fit.

INVOLVEMENT OF THE COMMUNITY IN PROMOTING PHYSICAL ACTIVITIES

Parents and teachers need to be encouraged to involve the community in promoting healthy development for children by planting in or creating more community gardens, participating in farmers' markets and community-supported agriculture, or sponsoring free sports and exercise classes for children.

In New York, the following are free for children:

- New York Junior Tennis & Learning
- Shape Up NYC
- New York City Department of Parks & Recreation
- Swim programs
- CityParks Kids

Physical exercise allows students to stay fit. Student athletes learn to become both mentally and physically prepared for life as a whole. Physical activity in basketball promotes healthy eating in order to maintain high performance and muscle recovery. When students have a proper diet plan they are able to perform well, remain fit, focused, and be consistent with their meal choices as they are educated on what helps them remain both physically and mentally prepared for practice and games.

Children need to be properly hydrated as well, especially when the outside temperature is high. Children should drink a lot of water, and should not be outside for an extended period in extreme conditions.

There are plenty of advertisements that showcase how athletes are able to perform well due to their determination to staying fit by exercising and making healthy food choices. Students learn not only from their environment but also their coaches. Coaches can empower children with the knowledge of how important healthy eating, exercising, and rest are to their success as student athletes.

Students who have positive figures in their lives gain the proper knowledge to help them make good choices pertaining to a healthy lifestyle, whether it is a coach mentioning how to build strength or a parent explaining the importance of eating healthy food to grow strong. Students seek answers and direction so it is the duty of parents, teachers, and society to help children understand why they should monitor their food intake, exercise, and sleep patterns. It is as important to stretch before beginning a workout as it is to eat high-protein foods to keep their bodies game-ready.

Coaches aim to help children build their stamina and allow them to perform at a high level and work through fatigue. Most importantly they have a team chef who helps student athletes plan their daily food intake and teaches them how to build muscle mass, and maintain a healthy heart and blood pressure. A team chef provides students with the opportunity to learn how eating right benefits their bodies and prepares them for life after being a part of the team.

It is important for adults to be mindful of how they approach situations when dealing with children. With the rapid growth in children, it is important that proper nutrition and health habits are stressed. Successfully meeting the challenges of children's nutrition requires collaboration among parents, teachers and other school personnel, key community members, registered dieticians, health-care providers, researchers, policy makers, and children themselves.

RECOMMENDATIONS ON WAYS TO INCORPORATE SPORTS AND PHYSICAL ACTIVITY TO HELP WITH PHYSICAL DEVELOPMENT

- Schools can offer a curriculum that includes health and science that explains the physical changes that adolescents are going through.
- Teachers can maximize activities where students work together more often so that they get to know each other.
- Teachers can design activities that help to build self-esteem by helping students to highlight things that they are good at doing.
- Teachers and school administration can work together to help to promote healthy eating habits.

DISCUSSION QUESTIONS

1. Why do you think physical exercise is important for young children?
2. How can sports, yoga, music, and dance contribute to the aspect of physical exercise among children?
3. List all the games and/or sports that children can be involved in inside the classroom and outside the classroom.

4. List all the games and/or sports for summer months and winter months.

REFERENCES

Abadie, B., and S. Brown. 2010. Physical activity promotes academic achievement and a healthy lifestyle when incorporated into early childhood education. *Forum on Public Policy* online 2010 (5).

Beighle, A., and F. Johnson. 2012. Increasing physical activity through recess. Research brief. Robert Wood Johnson Foundation.

Bergstein, C. D. 2010. Young children and movement: The power of creative dance. *National Association for the Education of Young Children* (March): 30–35.

Conklin, M. T., J. Marshak, and M. K. Meyer. 2004. The role of the school nutrition environment for promoting the health of young adolescents. *Middle School Journal* 35 (5) (May): 27–32. Retrieved from http://www.jstor.org/stable/23043718.

Dalton, S. 2013. Youth fitness: Exercise helps children excel in school. *Healthline* (October). Healthline Networks, Inc. Accessed May 7, 2015.

Datz, T. 2013. Poll finds lack of physical education in public schools a concern of parents. *Harvard T. H. Chan School of Public Health* (December). Retrieved from https://www.hsph.harvard.edu/news/press-releases/lack-of-physical-education-in-schools-concerns-parents/.

Dow, C. B. 2010. Young children and movement: The power of creative dance. *Young Children* 65 (2): 30–35.

Fisher, L. A., and M. N. Madeson. 2007. Put me in coach: The psychology of sports and physical activity for young adolescents. *The Young Adolescent and the Middle School*, 27–45. Retrieved from http://campusguides.stjohns.edu/ld.php?er_attachment_id=361338.

Golubovic, S., J. Maksimovic, B. Golubovic, and N. Glumbic. 2012. Effects of exercise on physical fitness in children with intellectual disability. *Research in Developmental Disabilities: A Multidisciplinary Journal* 33 (2): 608–14.

Guha, S. Summer, 2015. Lending a helping hand: A school in India for children who are blind. *Childhood Explorer* 2(3): 25–28.

Massey-Stokes, M. 2002. Adolescent nutrition: Needs and recommendations for practice. *The Clearing House* 76 (6) (August): 286–91. Retrieved from http://www.jstor.org/stable/30189764.

Motta, R. W., M. E. McWilliams, J. T. Schwartz, and R. S. Cavera. 2012. The role of exercise in reducing childhood and adolescent PTSD, anxiety, and depression. *Journal of Applied School Psychology* 28 (3): 224–38. Retrieved from http://www.tandfonline.com/doi/abs/10.1080/15377903.2012.695765?src=recsys&journalCode=wapp20.

4

SOCIAL AND EMOTIONAL CHALLENGES FOR CHILDREN WITH HEALTH ISSUES

LEARNING OBJECTIVES

1. How do children with health issues suffer socially?
2. How do children with health issues suffer emotionally?

Children's personality traits have been associated with their weight according to pediatric obesity studies conducted by the National Institutes of Health. More specifically, it has been found that in relation to their classmates of normal weight, overweight children have lower energy, concentration, optimism, compliance, perseverance, and self-confidence levels. At the same time, they have higher levels of egocentricity, irritability, and anxiety.

Another study has found that obese children suffer from high levels of loneliness. Even later in life, the image they retain about themselves is that of a troublemaker, of being sad, fearful, and wimpy (Rimm, 2004).

One of the most immediate and most difficult side effects children with obesity face is the stigmatization associated with obesity. Children with health issues such as obesity are more likely to suffer from a variety of social and emotional challenges than their peers. One of these is low self-esteem. Obese children look different than the average child because they weigh more. Due to their weight issues, peers may tease and ridicule them, augmenting their feelings of low self-esteem.

Children of normal weight tend to associate overweight children with negative characteristics such as laziness, lying, cheating, ugliness, and stupidity (Lobstein, Baur & Uauy, 2004). In one study, children were presented with various drawings of children with handicaps, including those who used crutches or were wheelchair-bound, were missing a limb or other significant body part, had a facial disfigurement, and were obese. Based on the ranking of what children "liked best," the children with obesity were ranked lowest (Strauss & Pollack, 2001). With this stigmatization, it is no wonder that children with obesity struggle with their self-esteem. Children with low self-esteem issues may lack personal friendships with peers.

The social stigma attached to being overweight can be as damaging to a child as the physical diseases and conditions that often accompany obesity. In a society that puts a premium on thinness, studies show that children as young as six years old may associate negative stereotypes with excess weight and believe that a heavy child is simply less likable (healthychildren.org).

The *International Journal of Obesity* conducted a study to determine if there is a causal relationship between young children of higher body mass index and young children with self-esteem issues. The study was conducted in elementary schools in Victoria, Australia, with a random sampling of children ages five years through ten years old. Researchers concluded "increasingly strong associations between lower self-esteem and higher body mass across the elementary school years" (Hesketh et al., 2004).

This association between body mass index (BMI) and self-esteem shows children with obesity are likely to face low self-image issues and should be monitored in order to prevent increasing emotional problems in their older years.

According to the International Association for the Study of Obesity, self-esteem issues associated with obesity may result in negative behaviors, such as unhealthy eating habits. For adolescents, the effects of a lack of self-esteem due to health issues can cause feelings of hopelessness and sometimes lead to suicide attempts. Many studies found that low self-esteem issues and dissatisfaction with the body are more commonly found in girls.

Children with health issues often suffer from low self-esteem because they feel bad about the way they look and feel. They worry about what other people think of them. They feel worthless and disgusted about themselves. They compare themselves to other children their age and are saddened by the fact that they are unable to function the way healthy children do. Stigmas are oftentimes attached to these children as well. Their physical talents are overlooked because of their weight or lack of physical activity. It is assumed that they cannot keep up or are unable to do what healthy children can do.

Bullying can also become a huge issue for children with health issues. In many cases these children are bullied by their peers and sometimes even by adults. They are called names or told that they are unable to do what a "normal" child can do. Fox and Farrow (2009) suggest that being overweight or obese is a risk factor for bullying and peer victimization. Obese children were more likely to be overt victims of bullying, compared to average-weight children. Unfortunately, these children can often become bullies themselves. Their self-esteem is so low that they try to make themselves feel better by putting other people down.

Dalton (2004) explores both the physical and psychological long-term effects that stem from childhood obesity. According to her book, a male who reaches a BMI of 45 in his twenties may actually cut his life span down by thirteen to twenty years. Obesity has also been connected to fatty liver disease, menstrual irregularities, and headaches among adolescents (Dalton, 2004).

The negative repercussions aren't only physical; there are many psychological problems that overweight children face. Pediatric youth research experts point out that obese children are often targets of discrimination. Further, low self-esteem puts overweight children at a higher risk for drug and alcohol abuse.

IMPACT OF ADVERTISING ON CHILDREN'S EMOTIONAL HEALTH

Food industry advertising that targets children and youth has been linked to the increase of childhood obesity. Advertising by other industries often objectifies girls and women, contributing to body dissatisfaction, eating disorders, low self-esteem, and depression. Many adolescents, particularly teenage girls, have body-image concerns and engage in unhealthy weight-control behaviors. Unhealthy weight-control behaviors (for example, fasting, skipping meals, eating very little food, vomiting, and using diet pills, laxatives, or diuretics) have been found to co-occur with obesity. Again media plays a big role here and teenage girls often feel so depressed that they try to take their own lives.

Weight bias may marginalize children and youth considered obese by their peers and teachers and place them at risk for teasing and bullying. Body dissatisfaction and weight-related concerns extend across all ethnic groups and weight-related stigma has been found to co-occur with depression, low self-esteem, and suicidal thoughts.

Following are excerpts from interviews with individuals who struggled with weight, but all of them agreed that losing weight didn't change the way they viewed themselves. They each mentioned that they felt like they would always be obese in their minds.

Jack, a young man, said that for him being overweight made him feel terrible about himself. He found himself being mean to other students during high school as a way to defend himself from the ridicule before it happened. High school for him was a time of feeling very alone, especially when it came to dating. Once he was in college and got gastric bypass surgery, he said people treated him completely different.

Women, in particular, were more likely to talk to him, but he was still insecure about all the extra skin left by the weight loss. He has since had the extra skin removed, but said that in his head, he still feels like he is 350 lbs., and he worries that those feelings of insecurity will never go away. It's been five years since his surgery, and he still finds himself questioning whether people who now speak to him would still be his friend if he was overweight.

Another man, Phillip, said that he struggled with weight issues his entire life. He found himself being made fun of in elementary school, and was often hesitant to participate in gym, because he couldn't keep up with the other kids, and often had trouble breathing. As he got into middle school the ridicule started, and he spent most of adolescence feeling isolated and alone. Once in high school, he realized that he could be accepted as the "party guy," and drugs and alcohol became a problem that he's battled with most of his life.

Sarah, a young woman suffered from an eating disorder all through high school. She was about forty pounds overweight, and even though she was starving herself most of the time, never lost much weight. Being an overweight female in high school meant she felt ostracized from her peers, especially the more "popular" groups of girls, who never wanted anything to do with her. She said she felt girls always had a tendency to be outwardly crueler to her than the boys.

Once in college, she sought help for her disorder, but even then, she said she felt alone, because her eating disorder didn't render her stick skinny. She often felt alone during her group therapy, and like she wasn't taken seriously when she disclosed her disorder to her friends and family. Years later, even at a healthy weight, Sarah struggles with viewing herself as over-weight.

The one thing that all three people interviewed seemed to share was that they felt alone and judged by their peers based on their weight. It was as if who they were as people didn't matter because nobody was looking past their physical appearance.

This is a problem that many obese people face. The Obesity Society has an entire section of their website (obesity.org, 2016) dedicated to the stereotypes and stigmas that obese people face every day, including verbal ridicule or being pointed out and laughed at in public. They often face embarrassing problems, like not being able to fit in certain seats, or finding that most medical equipment is too small for them.

According to both the Obesity Society website and from a study that Dalton (2004) mentions in her book, many health-care profes-sionals have an "implicit anti-fat bias" and show a tendency to "treat obesity" but associated obese people with "bad" and thin people with "good." Studies indicate that many health-care profes-sionals view those suffering with obesity as weak-willed, lazy, and lacking self-control (Dalton, 2004). Unfortunately, many obese people often find themselves facing work-related discrimination, as studies show they are less likely to be hired or are given lower wages.

Self-awareness about size and weight starts at a fairly early age, especially with female children. The media is full of images of what the "ideal body" shape is for both genders, and that can often put a lot of pressure on children and adolescents to look a certain way.

In a dance class, I was surprised to hear a five-year-old girl ask her mother if she was skinny. The mother was quite surprised at her daughter's concern. Later, the dance instructor explained that some of the girls in her dance class, ranging from five to nine years old, were worried that they were getting fat.

When I spoke to the dance instructor, she informed me that discussions about weight were fairly common at this age and that she had actually lost a few students who became self-conscious about their size and were uncomfortable wearing the leotards to class.

It's hard to imagine that anyone would judge a child based on weight, but according to a study (Dalton, 2004), when a group of children and adults were asked to rate six pictures of children with disabilities in order from those they felt they would like most to least, everyone in the study picked the obese child last. This study was later replicated by Latner and Stunkard (2003) where they took 458 fifth and sixth graders, ranging from upper-middle- to lower-middle-income families, and again found that students judged the obese child more harshly.

CHILDREN WITH WEIGHT ISSUES BECOME VICTIMS OF BULLIES OR BULLIES

In addition to the self-inflicted criticism and the struggle to lose weight, children with obesity face teasing and bullying. Teasing at school can cause a child with obesity to lose friends and avoid school. Bullying involves intentionally harming and repeating negative actions toward another child. Bullying can be verbal or physical, direct or indirect. Children who are bullied can suffer delays in cognitive or social development, lack of self-esteem, and even physical harm.

Research indicates children with obesity who are bullied are more likely to skip class and some eventually drop out of school. In an article published by *U.S. News & World Report*, *HealthDay* reporter Serena Gordon investigated children with obesity as a target for bullies. She reports that in a study at the University of Michigan in Ann Arbor, obesity "trumps [gender, race, and family income] when it comes to aggressive behavior from other children."

Researchers found that despite any other characteristics a child may have, it did not matter. Children with obesity are simply "more likely to be bullied." This research indicates a need to change the stigma associated with bullying in order to prevent the negative consequences of obesity that children face, especially self-esteem and peer bullying.

Children who are overweight are often bullied or made fun of in school. They have very low self-confidence, and they are not happy with the way they look. "Overweight children and teens who are bullied are often called names, punched, teased, ganged up on, humiliated and ignored relentlessly either in-person or in social media by mean and often troubled peers. Victims often feel depressed, sad, lonely, alienated, ostracized, angry, powerless, anxious and fearful" (obesityaction.org). These emotions can make going to school very hard for a child who is overweight, since many of them suffer from anxiety or depression.

It is imperative that we address bullying in our schools, neighborhoods, and communities because every child has the basic human right to feel safe and secure" (obesityaction.org). Bullying can traumatize a child. The public needs to become educated about the dangers of bullying and work as a community to identify and prevent instances of bullying.

Parents may schedule meetings with principals and counselors, and other school personnel may be trained to identify dangerous situations. It is important to listen to a child who has been the victim of bullying, and to come up with solutions that they are comfortable with.

One young man, stated: "Being obese I felt my high school years were brutal. I remember always being teased, called names like 'fatty' or 'porky' since as far back as I can remember. At first yeah it felt bad, no one likes to be teased, but I was very young—like five—so my close friends didn't really care if I was overweight. But as I got older friends and peers started judging who they wanted to be friends with, and it was rarely ever the fat kid. So finding friends was always tough and on top of that the bullies in school [preyed] on kids like me—the fat kid with no friends. I got teased a lot all throughout elementary and middle school."

I asked, "So how did all of that teasing and lack of friends impact your outlook on life, family life, and hope for the future?"

He said, "I got as sad and depressed as any young kid can get. I remember being 10 years old crying myself to sleep because I hated being so fat, I remember being filled up with so much anger. Anger towards my parents and my family for feeding me so much, sometimes I'd want to hurt myself or other people, but I guess I never lost hope. I often used to make fun of myself so I [could] make other kids laugh to feel accepted. I used to be the class clown but as I look back at it now I think it was just a defense mechanism of some sort. But I always knew one way or another I was going to lose the weight."

"And what made you think that?" I asked.

He said "Not sure. I was always a kid up for a challenge so maybe that combined with the fact that I was sick and tired of being treated like an outsider made me realize I can do something about it."

He continued by saying, "Once I started exercising and playing more sports, I saw some of the weight come off, that's when I got really motivated because I saw progress not only physically but socially as well. More sports outside meant I was interacting with more people and I actually made friends so that even motivated me more to continue to play sports and lose the weight. The rest of the weight kind of took care of itself once I hit my growth spurt."

I then asked, "Looking back at your childhood do you think there was anything your family, school, or community could have done to prevent your obesity?"

"Maybe," he said, "I guess my parents could have cooked more nutritious foods and watched my portions strictly. As far as school, that's tough because the food they served was fine but I guess if my classmates were more supportive, I know that's asking a lot from young kids but if kids can encourage other kids I feel like that's something that could have definitely helped me out."

"What about the community?" I asked.

He said, "Well as a young kid, I only knew about my community based on where and how often I visited these places with my family. My parents settled for fast food a lot, we were always at a drive-thru but at least my community where I grew up was an active one. I lived across the street from a park so there was always opportunities for active play."

In conclusion, James said, "Once I lost the weight I always stuck up for the ones being bullied. Even now, any chance I get to speak to an overweight kid, I take it because I know what he or she is going through and I want to let them know that there is hope there is something they can do about it. I know the negative self-esteem they feel and I just want to do anything I can to empower them."

Childhood obesity clearly has detrimental consequences for self-esteem. James's experience is just one of many. In fact among all youth, obese Hispanic and Caucasian females demonstrate significantly lower levels of self-esteem by early adolescence. Furthermore, obese children with decreasing levels of self-esteem demonstrate significantly higher rates of sadness, loneliness, and nervousness. However, the question that has been posed before and continues to vex researchers is whether obesity leads to social problems (loneliness, sadness, etc.) or is it the other way around—emotional and other mental health issues such as depression help spur children to become overweight (Goodwin, 2011)? A similar question may be posed as to whether obesity leads to behavioral issues, or is it vice versa—are behavioral problems antecedents to obesity?

Strauss and Pollack (2001) stated obese children are more likely to engage in high-risk behaviors such as drinking alcohol or smoking. In addition, children with ADHD symptoms are at an increased risk for becoming obese and physically inactive adolescents. Those results were yielded during a study that examined obesogenic behaviors to identify underlying ADHD symptoms. Although the author found correlating data, it was not arrived at in the manner predicted, which signifies to me a good starting point and a need for more research.

Pediatricians on the *Healthy Children* website give parents the following tips when dealing with bullying:

HOW PARENTS AND CHILDREN SHOULD RESPOND TO BULLYING

1. Tell an adult.
2. Stay in a group.
3. Do not react to the taunting because if the bully sees the victim becoming anxious or even start to cry, the teasing is likely to get worse. Encourage your child to maintain her composure, turn around, and walk away.
4. If the bullying continues, *only* if the victim feels safe, try being assertive and stand up to the tormentor. In some cases, a firm statement will neutralize the confrontation—something like "Stop bugging me!" The bully might react by turning his or her attention toward finding an "easier prey"—someone who doesn't fight back or appears more vulnerable to verbal attacks.
5. Let your child's teacher know about the harassment being directed at your youngster. The teacher may be able to intervene to put an end to it. If the teasing continues, ask the

school principal or your child's school counselor to get involved. Your youngster may be embarrassed to have you talk to the principal, but you can't afford to let her be mistreated any further. In fact, many schools now have anti-bullying policies. It is generally better to let the teacher and principal handle the situation, rather than to try contacting the bully or the bully's parents yourself.

6. Convince your child to try bonding more closely with the friends that he or she does have at school. If he or she hangs out with a group on the playground or in the lunchroom, she is less likely to be singled out for mistreatment.

7. Add an activity outside of school that the child can participate in, during which she can develop a new peer group that may be less inclined to tease. Sign up for a martial arts class or the Boy or Girl Scouts. These clubs help boost self-confidence.

8. Spend time with your child and treat him or her as an important person. Help maintain your child's self-esteem by demonstrating respect and acceptance and conveying the message, "I believe in you."

Source: healthychildren.org

Regrettably, obese children are about 65 percent more likely to fall victim to bullying than their normal-weight classmates (Lumeng, 2010). Even in cases where obese children possess qualities that would be typically viewed as likely to discourage bullies, such as having good social skills or doing well in school, they are still bullied more often than their normal-weight classmates.

Bullying of obese children has also been linked to the fact that most obese children suffer from low self-esteem, which makes them easier targets (Rimm, 2004). This phenomenon can be explained by the fact that, through their behavior, children are modeling respect for others based on weight.

Interestingly, studies have suggested that obese children are more likely to bully others, in addition to being the victims of bullying, mainly due to their difficulty remaining calm and controlling their impulses (Lumeng, 2010).

Bullying and "fat-shaming" behaviors do not encourage children to lose weight. Quite the opposite; they have negative effects on children suffering from obesity and can result in further weight gain, as children are caught in a vicious circle of self-destructive behavior (Rimm, 2004.). Even without bullying, inactivity and low self-esteem pushes obese children to use eating as a means to feel better. Bullying further intensifies this highly emotional and painful cycle.

The psychological stress of social stigmatization can cause low self-esteem, hopelessness, and discouragement in children. Children have a keen desire to feel and know that they are loved and accepted; bullying and social stigmatization interfere with their self-esteem, subsequently causing them to lack the ability to act independently, handle both positive and negative emotions, and handle peer pressure appropriately. Children who lack self-esteem are also less socially adept, which can create challenges for them when they are faced with or placed in social environments.

According to the Olweus Bully Prevention Program, there are nine different types of bullying. These include verbal bullying, social exclusion or isolation, physical bullying, bullying through lies and false rumors, having money or other things taken or damaged, being threatened or forced to do things, racial bullying, sexual bullying, and cyber bullying (via cell phone or the Internet).

All types of bullying need to be taken into consideration and need to be handled differently. Teachers, parents, educators, counselors, and administrators should be aware of these types of bullying and should be prepared to influence their children to not act in these ways.

HOW A CHILD WITH WEIGHT ISSUES FACES PRESSURE FROM PEERS

Children with health issues suffer from lack of self-esteem because they do not feel accepted or "equal" or similar to the rest of the people within their community or society. Oftentimes, these children are victimized by bullies because of their condition or their physical appearance.

A child who is obese is more likely to have low self-esteem than others. Weak self-esteem can translate into feelings of shame about their body, and lack of self-confidence can lead to poorer academic performance at school. These youngsters may be told by classmates (and even adults) that being heavy is their own fault. They might be called names. They could be subjected to teasing and bullying. Their former friends may avoid them, and they may also have trouble making new friends.

CASE STUDY

Michelle, age 7, was bullied in school by her classmates. She had weight issues. She was allergic to food with protein. Ever since birth, she had to maintain a very strict diet without protein. She was able to consume healthy foods that contained small amounts of protein as long as she was sure to drink or eat her medicine to balance the intake of protein levels; not following the strict diet caused health complications such as intellectual disability, seizures, and behavior problems, etc.

She has always been a little heavier than her brother; because of her treatment, however, she was not overweight because she was closely monitored as a child. Regardless, Michelle struggled with feeling out of place because she had weight issues. Recently, Michelle expressed that she was bullied as a child due to her condition. She stated that other children would see her eating her medicinal bar in class and they would make fun of her; they would make hurtful comments, point and say that she was eating "disgusting bars." This lowered her self-esteem significantly.

There was a period of time where she refused to tell anyone including friends about her condition because she was afraid of not being accepted. Students in her class would make fun of her physical appearance which has affected her till the present moment. She currently struggles with feeling good about herself physically and mentally due to her weight and acknowledgment of her condition. She received counseling from her dietician and nutritionist as they educated her more about her condition; the bullying of her childhood peers has still stigmatized her throughout her life.

Stevelos (2010) states that overweight children who are bullied are often called names, punched, teased, ganged up on, humiliated, and ignored. These awful things can happen to obese children in person or on social media. She states, "Victims often feel depressed, sad, lonely, alienated, ostracized, angry, powerless, anxious and fearful."

Stevelos (2010) shares in her article that in a "national survey of overweight sixth graders, 24 percent of the boys and 30 percent of the girls experienced daily teasing, bullying or rejection because of their size." These numbers double for overweight high school students.

It is important that we address the struggles of obese children. Changes must be made to better our schools, neighborhoods, and communities. It is really important to recognize that every child has the basic human right to feel safe and secure.

SOCIAL AND EMOTIONAL CHALLENGES: DEPRESSION

Another social and emotional challenge linked to childhood obesity is depression. Depression may occur because of self-hate or low self-esteem. Obese children may hate their appearance and feel horrible about themselves because they feel helpless about their weight. Being bullied in school, children with obesity issues may also be teased relentlessly about their weight, which can also lead to depression.

There is a correlation between overweight or obese children and the presence of depression and/or anxiety. Children who are over-weight more often suffer from emotional disorders. As children become more depressed or anxious, weight again continues, creating a vicious cycle. Both boys and girls suffer alike, although girls may suffer from more depression more frequently than boys (Rofey et al., 2009).

The challenges obese children face are not limited to emotional issues but include development delays as well, particularly in motor skills. Obese children show a significant lack of coordination skills. In particular, balance can be difficult for children who are obese. Overweight children also show a lack of competence in comparison to their peers who are not considered overweight. Young children feel inadequate and remove themselves from participating in physical activity which further contributes to the issue (D'Hondt, Deforche, De Bourdeaudhuij, & Lenoir, 2009).

Young children with weight issues can also develop a withdrawal syndrome from their peers. Research shows young children are being increasingly victimized by others because of their weight. They are mocked and bullied and referred to as dumb, lacking in self-control, and worthless. Not only peers, but also teachers and even parents often share this view.

The name-calling and labeling of young children as "fat" begins early and continues into adulthood. Many children who experience such bullying use food as comfort, augmenting the problem rather than finding a solution. Again physical education is the greatest tool to help children feel more confident and break the bad habits of obesity (Bromfield, 2009).

With all of this turmoil in overweight children's lives, they may feel as though they don't belong or fit in anywhere; they may see themselves as different or outcast. An overweight child often feels lonely and is less likely than his peers to describe himself as popular or cool. And when this scenario becomes ingrained as part of his life—month after month, year after year—he can become sad, clinically depressed, and withdrawn.

Schools across the globe should create anti-bullying teams, as well as provide workshops for students to collaborate with their peers on how to stop bullying. This will help break down social barriers by having students participate in ways to help improve their school and ultimately the world they live in. These little steps have huge effects and will help promote a positive social environment for children.

Fortunately, shortly after Oprah Winfrey announced the need for a national conversation on how to stop bullying in schools, a national campaign to stop bullying was started in 2010. Winfrey paved the way with her support in the fight against bullying. Now the month of October has been declared as "National Bullying Prevention Month." I feel if we all work on helping students understand how to love one another, then we can begin to build a safe environment for each student. My goals as a teacher are to help students remain safe, to provide them with knowledge, and to support them in their learning journey.

CULTURAL CONNOTATIONS ABOUT CHILDREN WITH HEALTH ISSUES

Negative connotations about being overweight and obese are not a global perspective. In some cultures, such as the Mexican culture (Gavin, 2014), being overweight is regarded as healthy and being well-cared for. These children do not face the effects of stigma, psychological problems, or peer rejection more than their peers of a normal weight. Based on these observations, it can be concluded that environmental factors impact the social and emotional effects of obesity.

DISCUSSION QUESTIONS

1. How do children with health issues suffer socially?
2. What can you do to help children who are suffering socially?
3. How do children with health issues suffer emotionally?
4. What can you do to help children who are suffering emotionally?
5. Explain how children with weight issues suffer from lack of self-esteem.
6. Explain how children with weight issues suffer from depression.
7. Explain how children with weight issues are bullied.
8. Explain how children with weight issues suffer academically.

REFERENCES

Bromfield, P. V. 2009. Childhood obesity: Psychosocial outcomes and the role of weight bias and stigma. *Educational Psychology in Practice* 25 (3): 193–209.

Dalton, S. 2004. *Our overweight children: What parents, schools, and communities can do to control the fatness epidemic.* Los Angeles: University of California Press.

D'Hondt, E., B. Deforche, I. De Bourdeaudhuij, and M. Lenoir. 2009. Relationship between motor skill and body mass index in 5- to 10-year-old children. *Adapted Physical Activity Quarterly* 26 (1): 21–37.

Fox, C. L., and C. V. Farrow. 2009. Global and physical self-esteem and body dissatisfaction as mediators of the relationship between weight status and being a victim of bullying. *Journal of Adolescence* 32 (5): 1287–301.

Gavin, M. L. 2014. Motivating kids to be active. *KidsHealth* (October).

Goodwin, J. 2011. Obese kids may face social, emotional woes. *Daily Health News* (September 21). https://www.rxshop.md/news/9637/.

Hesketh, K., M. Wake, and E. Waters. 2004. Body mass index and parent-reported self-esteem in elementary school children: Evidence for a causal relationship. *International Journal of Obesity* 28 (10): 1233–237.

Latner, J. D., and A. J. Stunkard. 2003. Getting worse: The stigmatization of obese children. *Obesity Research*, 11: 452–456. doi:10.1038/oby.2003.61.

Lobstein, T., L. Baur, and R. Uauy. 2004. Obesity in children and young people: A crisis in public health. *Obesity Reviews* 5 (S1) (May): 4–26.

Lumeng, J. 2010. Weight status as a predictor of being bullied in third through sixth grades. *Pediatrics* 125 (6) (June).

Rimm, S. 2004. New study ties obesity to bullying. *Bullying Recovery* (May 6). http://bullyingrecovery.org/2010/05/06/new-study-ties-obesity-to-bullying/.

Rofey, D. L., R. P. Kolko, A. M. Iosif, J. S. Silk, J. E. Bost, W. Feng, E. M. Szigethy, R. B. Noll, N. D. Ryan, and R. E. Dahl. 2009. A longitudinal study of childhood depression and anxiety in relation to weight gain. *Child Psychiatry and Human Development* 40 (4): 517–26.

Strauss, R. S., and H. A. Pollack. 2001. Epidemic increase in childhood over-weight, 1986–1998. *Journal of the American Medical Association* 286 (22): 2845.

Stevelos, J. 2010. Bullying, bullycide, and childhood obesity. *Obesity Action Coalition.* http://www.obesityaction.org/wp-content/uploads/Bullying-and-Bullycide.pdf.

WEBSITES

http://healthychildren.org
http://www.obesityaction.org

5

THE ROLES OF FAMILY AND SCHOOL IN PROVIDING NUTRITION EDUCATION FOR CHILDREN

LEARNING OBJECTIVES

1. How can educators and parents help children develop a healthy lifestyle?
2. How can teachers help families provide a nutritional education for their children?

Parents and teachers can be very influential in helping children to develop a healthy lifestyle. At a young age, the most powerful influence in a child's life is the primary caregiver. By establishing healthy eating habits at a young age, parents can avoid weight issues in later life.

Healthy eating habits start at home. Family plays a pivotal role in helping children become healthy adults. Children have a tendency to imitate what they see at home, and if their parents model healthy eating and exercise habits, these will become a part of that child's general routine.

I spoke with four parents, with children ranging from two to fifteen years of age, to discuss their views when it came to feeding their children. One mother, who has an eight-year-old son and fifteen-year-old daughter, expressed that she often felt that she could not properly provide nutritious meals for her children.

She works full-time, and does odds and ends to make extra money. She doesn't always have the time to cook and admitted that she often orders food in three to four times a week, usually pizza or Chinese food. Both of her children have been diagnosed as being obese, and her daughter suffers from asthma.

When she started losing weight herself, she changed the type of food she was buying, and she saw that her children also started to lose weight. She also started working out more, and saw that her daughter started to take more of an interest in working out with her. The daughter has told her mother that she is comfortable with her body and doesn't feel a need to be super skinny.

Ethnicity and culture play a large role in how weight is viewed. Studies show that while the rate of obesity is higher among African American and Hispanic or Latino adolescents, eating disorders are more common among Whites and Asians (Dalton, 2014). Genetics also play a large role in how our bodies store fat, and studies have shown that children who come from families with a history of weight issues are more likely to be overweight adults.

A study by Cardon (1994) explored a concept called adiposity rebound, which is the rapid accumulation of fat that occurs between the ages of 5.5–6.5 years and, depending on whether or not it occurs early, may be an indicator of future obesity. Having a child's BMI screened during this time may give parents a clue as to whether or not their children may be at risk (DeFries, Plomin, & Fulker, 1994).

Two of the other parents I spoke with had much younger children, both a little over the age of two. One father said that his son was a picky eater and that in order to get anything they could into him, they had started feeding him chicken nuggets, crackers, and dessert items. He said that during the first year of his son's life, the child had never been introduced to junk food, but it was all down-hill after the first birthday party, when his son discovered cake.

Another mother told me that her son also had never been introduced to junk food during his first year of life, but then started learning about it while being in daycare, and also when he was with grandparents. This mother said that at home she feeds him mainly organic homemade food, but she feels like there is only so much she can control when she isn't with him.

The third mother has an eight-year-old daughter who is very active in gymnastics. The child is in great physical condition, and mom said that she felt it was important for her daughter to be active because she is an overweight adult, and has always been on the heavier side. She didn't want her daughter to go through the same trials she faced. She also has a son who is fifteen years old, and is obese. She said that it is hard for him physically, but she feels like the social implications of obesity are harder on females, and she wanted to make sure her daughter never experienced what she did growing up.

When I interviewed a ten-year-old child who has weight issues, I started the interview by asking, "What is your favorite food?"

She told me she likes junk food such as McDonald's hamburgers, pizza, donuts, and fried foods. She seemed a little shy but when I asked whether she has any problems with socializing with her friends, she said "No." However, she knew that she was heavier than her friends and she said she recently tried to manage her weight by not eating too much junk food because she said she wants to look good like celebrities on TV.

When I visited her at her house, she wasn't physically active. Most of the time I was there, she watched TV or played with her phone except when her mom asked her to help her prepare for dinner. In my opinion, she didn't seem to have serious problems like those I've read about in some articles regarding social and emotional issues among obese children. Perhaps this is because she is not that much overweight, just a little chubbier than other kids around her age, and she said she gets along well with her friends.

It was good to see that she doesn't have depression nor socializing problems, but her mom said she was a little concerned because her daughter is not as active as she used to be and stays home more of the time, and she has tried to go on a diet, either starving herself or eating everything at once.

What can we do as a family unit to promote physical fitness and decrease the possibility of obesity? The answer seems to be to lead by example; eat and exercise as a family unit. If the children are young, parents can take them food shopping and have them pick out their own fruits and vegetables. If they are a little older, have them cook with you in the kitchen. Regardless of age, talk to them openly about making healthy decisions, and encourage them to go outside and play.

Allow them to try different physical activities to see which ones they like best. Look into what activities are happening at the local parks and libraries, and encourage them to get involved in any extracurricular activities that their schools may offer.

When encouraging your child to lose weight, you want to make sure that they are doing it in a physically and psychologically healthy manner. Studies have found that nearly half of girls in second grade report wanting to be thinner, and that an estimated 40 to 60 percent of high school–aged girls have been on a diet. An eating disorder is a dangerous condition, whether it involves binge eating or the severe restriction of caloric intake. It is hard to unravel the mind-set that goes into an eating disorder, and often those diagnosed with one will continue to feel uncomfortable about their appearance regardless of what others say.

The best way to handle this is to talk to your child about healthy weight loss. When you stop eating for a few days, the pounds that are dropped are water weight, but that lower number on the scale often works as a motivation to restrict more calories. However, in reality, this cycling of weight loss and gain is bad for metabolism; and the weight usually doesn't stay off for very long.

The healthiest way to lose weight is slowly through consistent exercise and a healthy nutritious diet. Kuffel (2013) discusses how she has struggled with obesity her entire life. She encourages parents of obese children and adolescents to read up on nutrition, binge eating disorder, and obesity. This way they can learn that sugary or processed food can be highly addictive.

She encourages parents to learn about healthy ways for their child to lose weight and to encourage them to get the daily caloric intake they need to grow. She explains how when she was fifteen years old, she cut her calories down to 500 per day, and exercised four hours a day; her parents thought it was great, but it was really unhealthy.

It is becoming clearer to researchers that food addiction is a real disorder. MRIs and PET scans have shown that nearly 90 percent of dopamine receptors in the brain are active during eating "hyperpalatable" foods. A study on rats showed that within a week of being on a high-fat diet, there was permanent scarring in the part of the brain that controls weight. This pattern also showed in the scans of obese people.

On top of eating together as a family and encouraging as much physical activity as possible, the author suggests that families can help their children lose weight in a healthy manner by keeping the house free of high-calorie snacks, keeping an eye out for signs of depression, encouraging their child to find clothes that flatter their figure, and always letting your child know that you love him or her, regardless of their weight (Kuffel, 2013).

THE ROLES OF PARENTS AND OTHER FAMILY MEMBERS

Parents and other family members play critical roles in providing nutrition and managing weight issues. Through the early stages of childhood development, parents need to oversee their child's eating habits and correct them when appropriate. Children often model the types of behaviors exhibited by their parents and that in and of itself should give parents incentive to "lead by example" through exhibiting nutritious-conscious behaviors and eating habits.

When caring for an obese child or if obesity affects more than one family member, making healthy eating and regular exercise a family activity can improve the chances of successful weight control for the child.

Other effective measures parents can take in order to manage obesity and provide nutritional insight include starting a weight management program; whether as a family or individually, starting a weight management program provides an outlined, set plan on how and when a weight goal will be accomplished. Parents can attempt to change eating habits during the early stages of childhood development when eating patterns are formed. Parents should encourage the child to eat slowly and to develop a routine.

Parents should also plan meals and make better food selections by eating less fatty foods and avoiding junk and fast foods. Planning meals provides parents with the opportunity to control portions and serving sizes and to decrease calories. Children should also be encouraged to increase physical activity.

Parents can do this by incorporating physical activity into family time, such as taking walks together, or by enrolling their child in extracurricular physical programs. Families should also encourage children to eat meals with the family instead of while watching TV or on the computer. Such a family meal environment allows parents to connect with their child who may need that open contact to vent about self-esteem or mental health issues.

Finally parents must limit snacking for their children. Children who snack throughout the day tend not to have a balanced diet. Encouraging children to limit snacks in favor of a main meal is healthy; it also makes mealtimes less stressful for the parent.

Children imitate what they see and hear. By eating healthy foods themselves, parents will promote good eating habits in their children. Encourage active playtime by establishing regular family activities such as walking, ball playing, riding a bicycle, and other outdoor activities. "Physical activity in children and youths is associated with health benefits, including lower levels of being overweight and obese" (Hills, Andersen, & Byrne, 2011).

Parents can also educate children in making healthy decisions on types of foods and beverages as well as controlling portion size. Parents can encourage healthful eating habits at home by increasing the number of family meals eaten together, making healthy foods available, and reducing the availability of sugar-sweetened beverages and sodas.

Studies indicate that eating dinner together as a family promotes healthful eating among children by increasing their consumption of fruits, vegetables, and whole grains and by reducing their consumption of fats and soft drinks (Lindsay et al., 2006).

Eating breakfast is another way for parents to help their children prevent obesity. Even if it's not a whole meal, just eating something light such as fruits, cereal, or a glass of milk will help children maintain their energy throughout the day without overeating during lunch. If you can get your kids to establish the habit of eating a good breakfast at a young age, it should stay with them as they get older.

"Although the quality of breakfast was variable within and between studies, children who reported eating breakfast on a consistent basis tended to have superior nutritional profiles than their breakfast-skipping peers. Breakfast eaters generally consumed more daily calories yet were less likely to be overweight. Breakfast consumption could impact cognitive performance by alleviating hunger and has been associated with emotional, behavioral, and academic achievement in children and adolescents. Breakfast may modulate the short-term metabolic responses of fasting conditions to maintain a supply of nutrients to the central nervous system, or through long-term effects on nutrient intake and status that may positively affect cognition" (Rampersaud et al., 2005).

I interviewed a mother of two children. To help her provide good nutritional habits, she said she searched how to help her achieve her weight goal and be a good model to her kids. I started the interview by asking, "What are some ways in which you inspire your daughter to eat healthy?"

First, she eliminated buying extra snacks such as chips or sweet cookies. Instead, she tries to buy and provide fruits for dessert after meals. She also tries to cook more often than before and is avoiding processed food for her children. She said she used to buy takeout foods for dinner a lot of the time after work when she was tired— pizza, fried foods, or something that was easy for her. Now she tries to cook herself and gets her kids involved in ways such as putting utensils on the table or letting them do some actual cooking, which she said her daughter enjoys a lot.

I asked, "What are some challenges of providing nutrition for your children?" First, changing the children's habit of eating junk food and eating outside food were hard because she believed that she wasn't the greatest cook. Her foods were a little more bland. Another challenge was to try to cook a full meal. She had to search for recipes and cook something for dinner after a long day of work.

Another mother of two is mindful of healthy food and offers healthy food at home. She has banned soda at home completely. She hopes her children get movement or exercise every day, because one day a week in the gym is not enough. She said that, in

Denmark, every hour or half hour, children get up and go some movement like jumping-jacks. This helps circulation and blood flow. Here, in the United States, there is more focus on academics and children sit for long hours. With pressure on academics, children are losing out on their development. Further, taking away recess as a punishment is not right at all! Academics ought to be coupled with exercise. This mother also mentioned that it is tough for working parents who come home late to create activities during the weekday, so, thankfully, after-school activities have taken up that part. What different community centers can do is, when parents drop off their kids, they can also have activities for parents so that they can be engaged as well, because parents are their children's role models. Taking classes with parents and kids at the same time is a great idea for after-school hours.

Yet another mother I spoke to had this to say:

I have minimized our son's sugar intake and allow very limited processed foods to teach him moderation.In the beginning, juice was watered down, and now at eight years old, he will always ask me for a glass of water. Not juice. Not soda. Just water. Since he is often with me grocery shopping, I teach him about seasonal vegetables, the benefits they have for our bodies and why our berries and spinach must be organic. I also teach him how to be mindful when eating cookies and candy. He knows that sugar makes him excited and jokes about it when he is overflowing with energy and asks for a snack. That said, when he is offered sweets, he often declines even if I say it is okay (I try to not be hard on him or judgemental, just honest with humor).

On a daily basis, my son will start his day with a bowl of Cheerios with hormone-free organic whole milk. Dinner is chicken nuggets with pasta, or chicken with Brussels sprouts. Black beans and rice is a staple, and he loves Chipotle. Our food is for the most part *clean*. Although chicken nuggets are processed to some extent, I always look for chemical-free ingredients on every package. If I cannot pronounce an ingredient, I don't buy it.

I keep an eye on my son's vegetable consumption and make sure he eats as many colors of plant-based foods as possible. Chicken is his usual protein. On occasion he will eat an organic vegan sausage. He knows he has to try new foods. He doesn't always like what he tries, but he knows that trying it is non-negotiable. He knows it's important. For example, I explain why, when I'm not feeling well or if he is not feeling well, that we eat organic broth or sea vegetables, and why we can't eat dairy. I can also heal stomach aches, colds, lower cholesterol, chronic illness, etc., with food.

I will admit, I don't monitor what he buys for lunch at school. I want him to learn how to independently make smart decisions without us. I will ask what he eats and it's usually peanut butter and jelly or a hamburger. He drinks chocolate milk daily. I'm not thrilled about this, but I suspect my son feels some peer pressure to eat certain things. I cannot worry about this because I'd prefer for him to focus on growing his personality and independence, since he is an only child.

My son goes to swim lessons for half-an-hour per week and is an excellent swimmer. He will come with me for two mile walks without issue and walks through NYC like anyone else who lives here. He is fortunate to have skinny genes and is quite lean and then, with trim muscle. I encourage him to try sports and we are currently looking into him joining a track team. My primary reason for encouraging more sports is not only for exercise but so he can learn the benefits of personal and team competition. I strongly feel this will help him as he gets older, so I hope we can find a track team for him to experience.

There are plenty of opportunities to get involved with the community to foster good health for him, as well as for other children. When Queens County Farm museum has their Farm Stand in season, we visit there weekly for fresh local and organic produce before going to the grocery store. He understands the veggies we see were grown on that farm down the road. He even tasted a rutabega and loved it! (This is why we try new things.)

As a community, it is imperative to make fresh, local and organic food available and TEACH the reasons for its importance to our environment, our finances, the impact on our planet, and the impact on our personal health. There are many misconceptions about food and big agriculture is a serious threat to our well-being, as well as not being regulated by a third-party or reputable part of our government to protect our society. This is why we have to get involved and why other parents should get involved, too.

There are many positive ways that parents can educate children about making healthy choices. Strategies to incorporate healthy eating at home can be found in the many resources available to parents. For example, *KidsHealth*'s online article "Healthy Eating" suggests regular family meals, serving a variety of healthy food and snacks, acting as a role model, avoiding battles over food, and involving kids in the process. These tips apply to any household, as they are simple and manageable for the families who have busy lifestyles (Gavin, 2014).

Additionally, parents can educate themselves on healthy food choices and the economical options available to provide children with nutritious food. From the perspective of a school nurse, parents are to be held accountable because they often provide children with food and snacks that only exacerbate the problem.

The environmental factors that play a role in food selection, such as socioeconomic status, can negatively affect a child's perception of healthy eating. Families buy the less expensive and less nutritious food because it is what they can afford. However, families need to be made aware that there are healthy food choices they can make with the same monetary value.

While parent(s) are a child's primary educator, nutritional education should not end in the home. Educating children on healthy lifestyle choices is an essential aspect of their intellectual and physical development. Teachers, school nurses, and coaches have a responsibility to teach children about the consequences of their choices in foods and behaviors.

In the wake of the obesity epidemic, there is evidence of nutritional education efforts in schools. For example, the MyPlate initiative funded by the US Department of Agriculture is a program that is aimed at the current school-age population through the use of technology. The program's platform, ChooseMyPlate (https://choosemyplate.gov), is a website for children to access and learn about how to choose healthy meals in an interactive way.

As stated on the website, MyPlate provides practical information to help the population "build healthier diets with resources and tools for dietary assessment, nutrition education, and other user-friendly nutritional information." In relation to the obesity epidemic, MyPlate "empower[s] people to make healthier food choices for themselves, their families, and their children" (US Department of Agriculture).

Research suggests that schools can play a key role in the prevention of obesity through the implementation of strategies that promote health. To provide the necessary support, schools should first develop and introduce nutritional lessons and programs within the school curriculum. Emphasis on the importance of balanced and healthy nutrition should be incorporated as a separate subject, but also through other subjects such as science, chemistry, mathematics, and English.

A variety of nutrition books that teachers can base their lesson on are available. Educators can include these in their curriculum lesson plans connected with health and nutrition, and can also provide books to children's families to read in order to adopt healthy habits in the home environment.

Another measure that schools have been required to adopt within the United States is the banning of junk food within schools. The US Department of Agriculture has issued new rules toward combating obesity. Items that are sold in schools cannot contain more than 35 percent sugar or fat, while only water, low-fat and no-fat milk, and 100 percent fruit or vegetable juices are allowed as beverages. Vending machines are only allowed to sell fruit, dairy products, whole-grain foods, lean-protein products, or vegetable items that are less than 200 calories for "snacks" and 350 calories for main dishes.

There are several things that parents and schools can do to keep kids healthy. First and foremost, both parents and schools should be providing nutritious food to the children. In an article published on young children's eating behaviors, Eliassen (2011) emphasizes the impact that educators can have on their students' eating habits. She says that, "Early childhood educators who understand the importance of their role in the development of children's healthful eating behaviors can help improve the lifelong health of the children they serve. They can offer meaningful, positive experiences with food, including growing, preparing, and eating foods with children."

Regardless of the food offered at home, the early childhood educator has the opportunity to model selection and enjoyment of a variety of foods. This points to the idea that even if children are not being fed properly at home, teachers can still have an enormous impact on what the children eat.

Schools are trying to take active measures to prevent the obesity epidemic. Although there are posters hanging in school hallways that promote healthy eating and classrooms have lessons that incorporate information on food groups, the prevalence of obesity in young children has not been curtailed by these efforts.

Although the school menu designed by a nutritionist is a positive step in the movement to promote healthy eating, unfortunately there are still some unhealthy snack choices. Further, the food that is offered to the students may not be fresh. From the MyPlate initiative, schools can continue to promote healthy eating by incorporating nutritional education in curricula across all grade levels.

More visual aids and providing more physical education classes may be difficult for some schools in financial despair.

Nevertheless, while obesity remains of high concern, any and all positive changes should be considered, especially since some children with obesity have little opportunity to participate in physical activity. ChooseMyPlate can be used as a basis for a curricular unit. Teachers can incorporate MyPlate in math instruction through the use of visual aids such as graphs of food groups, numbers using nutrition labels, and measurement.

At school, students can practice their writing skills by sending letters to school authoritative figures petitioning for more opportunities for physical activity during the school day or by writing opinion pieces on the school food menu, they can read material that promotes healthy lifestyles, and they can conduct research projects, such as biographies, on individuals who lead healthy eating initiatives such as the one started by former first lady Michelle Obama. The US Department of Agriculture secretary released a new food icon called "MyPlate." This icon was created to remind people to make healthier food choices.

Created in an effort to battle childhood obesity across the nation, the Let's Move! initiative, also launched by Michelle Obama, seeks to provide parents with information and to develop environments to support healthy choices. The ultimate goal is to have a healthy future for our children.

Other school instruction could include an art activity to design a lunchbox using the MyPlate food group sections, dancing during music class for extra kinesthetic activity, and exploring the ChooseMyPlate (https://choosemyplate.gov) website during computer instruction. The possibilities are countless, helping teachers to provide children with nutritional education.

One effective way of motivating children is to create an environment where children learn to feel good about themselves. For instance, you could introduce children to different hobbies, sports, and neighborhood activities. Encourage them to pursue what they enjoy, and help children recognize that taking care of their bodies allows them to do what they like to do while maintaining limits on the amount of time spent watching TV and playing computer games. Make sure to turn off the TV during meals and when no one is watching it.

INPUT FROM EXPERTS: THE DIETICIAN OR NUTRITIONIST IN THE FIELD

Children can lead healthy lifestyles by eating healthy, being active, and exercising. Children should eat a variety of foods from the five food groups. This way they get all the essential nutrients they need. Children should be taught how to select food and beverages and what to look for while shopping. Most importantly, children should eat protein, whole grains, vegetables, and fruits, and reduce their sugar and sodium intake. Children can be encouraged to eat healthy food through parental influence.

Parents can provide a healthy breakfast with fiber, fruit, and dairy to start their child's day off right. Pack the child's school lunch making sure it contains food from the five food groups as much as possible, and provide natural and organic food. For children who are overweight, instead of a strict diet, it is better to make simple changes that have a larger overall impact on the child's poor habits. It is important to make a positive food relationship for children to avoid struggles and stress.

If parents model a healthy lifestyle and set a good example, children will likely follow in their footsteps. Parents can encourage their children to exercise by exercising with them as a family. Parents can also encourage outdoor play and sports. Parents can take children to sports events and find out what they are interested in.

Students should always choose physical activity over sedentary activity. Any type of daily physical activity is recommended. Some great physical activities for children are karate and yoga. Children should also get between eight and sixteen hours of sleep a day, depending on their age.

It is evident schools, teachers, nurses, and communities need to work together to help promote healthy eating habits so everyone can begin to live a healthier lifestyle. According to one nurse, when a child is diagnosed as obese, stress tests are conducted. The child runs on a treadmill with oxygen and the nurse monitors how the heart works daily. The nurse said that they then treat each patient as though they are diabetic because, unfortunately, many obese children are likely to develop type 2 diabetes over time.

The nurse stated that parents are required to do certain things after consultation with the nurse and are always referred to a nutritionist so they may develop a meal plan based on the child's BMI. After the parents and child meet with the nutritionist, they then see a psychologist to discuss how to make major changes in the child's life.

A pediatric physician's assistant was interviewed and provided many insights on childhood obesity. She suggests emphasizing the importance of a healthy diet to parents of children who already have obesity or display habits that can lead to obesity with time. Many parents are unaware of the long-term implications of childhood obesity; inform parents that a child will carry healthy nutrition and exercise habits with them into the future when they reach adulthood.

Children form lifestyle habits at an early age. Parents should address these issues when children are young and teach them healthy eating and exercise habits. It is definitely important to include the child in making healthier lifestyle choices; then it becomes a family experience.

A school nurse shared some simple and important ways educators and parents can help children to develop healthy habits. As a first step, overweight and obese patients and their families can focus on basic healthy lifestyle eating and activity habits. She also sends home a handout about maintaining a healthy lifestyle.

Nurses can help provide families with nutrition education for their children. School nurses provide skilled nursing services to students with documented needs. Referrals are sent to parents and guardians if further assessment is needed. Nurses provide ongoing case management for students with identified acute and chronic health problems (for example, obesity) to confirm that students are receiving prescribed services.

School nurses also implement the Healthy Options for Physical Activity and Nutrition Program (HOP'N) to assist children and families in developing healthy lifestyles. Nurses provide families of students with a body mass index (BMI) greater than the 99th percentile with clinical assessment, health education, counseling, and referrals to available resources in the community.

The nurse expressed how a lot of families are unaware and do not have the mental capacity to understand how detrimental high sugar, saturated fats, genetically modified ingredients, fried foods, and artificial ingredients are to their children's health.

In order to help parents understand how harmful these foods and ingredients are for their children, nurses take on the role of referring families to see a nutritionist so they may develop an individual meal plan (based on the body mass index) for each child. After the child visits the nutritionist, he or she is referred to a psychologist. The psychologist takes this opportunity to speak with the child about their feelings and thoughts as well as to help the child adapt to their proposed new lifestyle of eating healthy.

There are a lot of things that parents can do to keep their children healthy from the start. Pediatricians recommend that first of all a mother should have a healthy pregnancy. It is extremely important to take prenatal vitamins, avoid alcohol and caffeine, and maintain healthy exercise and sleep patterns. Pediatricians further recommend that mothers should nurse their babies if at all possible and as long as possible. They recommended keeping children active from the start.

They should be enjoying physical activities and learning to move their muscles. Children who are simply placed in front of a TV will not develop like those who are engaged in different sensory activities. As children grow older and learn to walk, they will naturally have a significant amount of energy if they are fed properly. They should be able to play and exercise their gross motor skills and engage in at least one hour of physical activity per day.

Parents need not only to transmit valuable information and knowledge about health but also to actively adopt a healthy lifestyle and thus become role models themselves. As children are dependent on their families to purchase and prepare their meals, steps such as adopting healthier cooking alternatives for traditional recipes and preparing healthy lunchboxes for the children to take with them to school can make a significant difference. In addition, through their home environment, children should be taught about mindful eating, appropriate portion sizes, and how to read nutrition labels.

In addition, parents and their children must get moving! They need to become more physically active. They can choose indoor or outdoor activities that they enjoy, so they become part of their daily routine. Together, they can have fun in other ways. Dance to your favorite music, walk the dog, take a class in martial arts, participate in sports, ride bike. Parents can walk their kids to school instead of driving. Also, they can take the stairs instead of the elevator. Parents must be the child's role model and must set good examples for the child.

Some families need a counselor for help with parenting skills, resolution of family conflict, or motivation. Parents must also follow up with specialists. A multidisciplinary team with experience in childhood obesity, including a behavioral counselor (social worker, psychologist), a registered dietician, an exercise specialist, and a primary care provider who continues to monitor medical issues and maintains a supportive alliance with families, should be involved. Educators can also reinforce these through classroom activities, gym, and extracurricular interests.

The ongoing epidemic of childhood obesity highlights the pressing need for serious lifestyle interventions. Family plays an essential role in influencing children to adopt a healthy and active lifestyle, and parents are usually critical role models when it comes to nutrition choices. Overall, there are three types of school involvement: at the minimal level, the school is the actor that tells, informs, and makes requests of the family; at the associate level, the school actively involves parents; and at the decision-making level, schools and families join their forces toward developing good learning opportunities for children (Comer et al., 1996).

Schools and parents have a huge influence on the health of children. By educating our children on healthy eating, we give them a foundation of knowledge that they can use for the rest of their lives. Although fast food might be easier and cheaper, it is very important to monitor the kind of connection we create between children and food.

Educators can offer a variety of healthy activities from which children can choose; acknowledging their accomplishments serves as positive reinforcement. Teachers can also include activities that students will most likely enjoy throughout their lifetimes.

Educators can inform parents of the unit themes that are being completed in class and encourage their involvement. Educators can send a letter home including a variety of activities for parents to complete in the home with their children. Educators can also educate parents on alternative strategies to implement in their daily routines.

It is most important to educate families on the importance of being active regardless of whether a child or a person has a health condition or not. The nurse stated that she encourages families to be a part of the activities instead of parents requesting their children to perform or complete physical activity. She indicated that she also encourages parents to include their children in extracurricular activities that they enjoy or to include other children and friends in the physical activities that they do together.

It is difficult as children get older for parents to be as involved in their lives. However, a parent's guidance is more influential than they presume. Consistency is crucial because healthy choices become healthy habits.

Childhood obesity is usually associated with eating junk, fatty food, overeating, and limited physical activity. Most children do not meet the nutritional and physical recommendations for a healthy lifestyle. There are many factors contributing to this. "The quality of available foods and beverages, means for physical activity, and patterns of sleep, as well as parental modeling and involvement, all influence childhood obesity" (Perryman & Sidoti, 2015). Food marketed toward children has been shifting toward foods with higher calories, higher fat, and higher sugar, such as fast food and sugar-based drinks.

Children's parents have a direct influence on the food they consume. "Some research shows that an authoritative parenting style decrease[s] the risk of obesity and increase[s] the amount of healthy food eaten when compared to other types of parenting. However, overly controlling feeding practices may negatively impact the child's food selections, as well as the amount of food consumed and eating frequency, consequently affecting the child's weight" (Perryman & Sidoti, 2015). A good practice that can help build nutritional knowledge for children is for parents to cultivate healthy nutrition and make physical activity a daily practice.

DISCUSSION QUESTIONS

1. How can educators and parents help children develop a healthy lifestyle?
2. How can teachers help families provide nutrition education for their children?

REFERENCES

Cardon, L. R. 1994. Height, weight, and obesity. In *Nature and nurture during middle childhood*, ed. J. C. DeFries, R. Plomin, and D. W. Fulker, 165–72. Cambridge, MA: Blackwell Publishers.

Comer, J. P., N. M. Haynes, E. T. Joyner, and M. Ben-Avie, eds. 1996. The school development program. In *Rallying up the whole village: The Comer process for reforming education*, 1–27. New York: Teachers College Press.

Dalton, S. 2004. *Our overweight children: What parents, schools, and communities can do to control the fatness epidemic*. Los Angeles: University of California Press.

DeFries, J. C., R. Plomin, and D. W. Fulker, eds. 1994. *Nature and nurture during middle childhood*. Cambridge, MA: Blackwell Publishers.

Eliassen, K. E. 2011. The impact of teachers and families on young children's eating behaviors. *Young Children* (March): 84–89.

Gavin, M. L. 2014. Motivating kids to be active. *KidsHealth* (October).

Hills, A. P., L. B. Andersen, and N. M. Byrne. 2011. Physical activity and obesity in children. *British Journal of Sports Medicine* 45 (11) (September): 866–70.

Kuffel, F. 2013. Don't talk to your overweight teen—act! The shame and pain of being an overweight teen. *Psychology Today* (June). Retrieved May 1, 2016, at http://www.psychologytoday.com/blog/what-fat-women-want.

Lindsay, A. C., K. M. Sussner, J. Kim, and S. Gortmaker. 2006. The role of parents in preventing childhood obesity. *Future Child* 16 (1) (Spring): 169–86.

Perryman, M. L., and K. A. Sidoti. 2015. Ethical considerations in the treatment of childhood obesity. *Dove Medical Press Ltd. UK* 2015 (5):17–26.

Rampersaud, G., M. Pereira, B. Girard, J. Adams, and J. Metzl. 2005. Breakfast habits, nutritional status, body weight, and academic performance in children and adolescents. *Journal of the American Dietetic Association* 105 (5) (June).

6

INVOLVEMENT OF THE COMMUNITY IN PROMOTING HEALTHY DEVELOPMENT FOR CHILDREN

LEARNING OBJECTIVES:

1. How would you encourage parents and teachers to involve the community in promoting overall healthy development for children?
2. What are some of the dance and sports programs in the community?
3. What are some of the types of food and restaurants that exist in the community?

An article entitled "Child Obesity: A Global Public Health Crisis" talks about ways in which we can help to get the "nutritious" word out. Community members can organize social events like healthy food festivals and harvest festivals, imparting healthy messages and encouraging people to change to or to continue with a healthy lifestyle. Also programs like providing playgroups with safe playgrounds and bike paths for kids to play outside will reduce the time they spend in front of the television.

A child is surrounded by home and family members, neighborhood, school, teachers, media, and culture. When families are supported, children are less likely to be at risk and more likely to grow up happy and healthy.

As far as the community food environment is concerned, in 2002 more than 35 million Americans experienced limited access to nutritious food on a regular basis (Institute of Medicine, 2005). Moreover, the availability of high-calorie, low-nutrient foods has increased in low-income neighborhoods due to many factors including supermarkets relocating to suburbs, consumers' lack of transportation to supermarkets, and the proliferation of convenience stores typically offering a limited selection of healthy foods at higher prices in these communities.

Some communities are improving food availability in a variety of ways such as offering grants, loans, and tax benefits to stimulate the development of neighborhood grocery stores in underserved urban neighborhoods. They are initiating farmers' markets, and promoting community gardens and farm-to-cafeteria programs.

Local governments should work with community groups, non-profit organizations, local farmers and food processors, and local businesses to support multispectral partnerships and networks that expand the availability of healthy foods within walking distance, particularly in low-income and underserved neighborhoods. Such efforts will expand healthy food options at local grocery stores, supermarkets, and fast-food restaurants, and they will encourage a broad range of community food security initiatives that improve access to healthy food.

Some of the community groups that can help to prevent childhood obesity are:

• Children, Youth, Parents, Families
• Child- and Youth-Centered Organizations
• Community-Based Organizations
• Community Development and Planning
• Employers and Work Sites

- Food and Beverage Industries, Food Producers, Advertisers, Marketers, and Retailers
- Foundations and Nonprofit Organizations
- Government Agencies and Programs
- Health- and Medical-Care Professional Societies
- Health-Care Delivery Systems
- Health-Care Insurers, Health Plans, and Quality Improvement and Accrediting Organizations
- Health-Care Providers
- Mass Media, Entertainment, Recreation, and Leisure Industries
- Public Health Professionals
- Recreation and Sports Enterprises
- Researchers
- Schools, Child Care Programs

In order for children to gain the motivation to be healthy, healthy lifestyles need to be promoted in the three main environments of a child's life: home, school, and community. For children to obtain the opportunity to succeed in making healthy lifestyle choices, there must be options for them to be active outside of school.

Parents and teachers can encourage the community in promoting overall healthy development for children by encouraging physical activity during out-of-school hours utilizing the facilities in the community. Parents and teachers can involve themselves in the intramural and sports activity clubs that are provided by the community.

Parents and teachers should encourage community members to promote consumer awareness when shopping for healthy food. Many healthy food choices do not have to be expensive. The community should provide more stores that sell healthy foods and advertise organic foods.

Beyond the immediate neighborhood, the greater community influences children through television, radio, magazine, and Internet advertisements that market unhealthy foods. By catering to children's preferences, food companies could influence children to reject unhealthy food choices. Marketing techniques are an environmental factor that affects children all over the world. Pressure needs to be applied at the national level to put restrictions on food companies so that they will not market foods to children that are high in fats, sugars, and salt.

Since media has a lot of influence on the children, healthy food should be advertised as a top priority and unhealthy food should be avoided. This will benefit children and help them build a positive self-image.

No matter how well parents promote healthy eating, it can be difficult for any kid to avoid the temptation of junk food. Instead of eliminating junk food entirely, which tends to increase cravings even more, try substituting some healthier alternatives.

Avoid sodas—children should drink water or milk instead. Avoid chicken nuggets—they are an unhealthy imposter of real chicken. Consider taking along a bag of mini carrots, grapes, or other fruits and vegetables to eat instead of French fries. Try chicken and vegetables or spaghetti with tomato sauce in a sit-down restaurant rather than a big plate of macaroni and cheese.

I interviewed a mother who was a waitress. Following is her quote:

> I was serving in a restaurant and I asked the customers if they want[ed] juice. They insisted they want[ed] punch and did not understand that punch has no fruit juice in it. Therefore, they need a lot of education. In school, they can teach home economics classes, for example, boiling [an] egg at home is not hard to learn, but [children] order food from restaurant[s] all the time. The amount of sugar, salt, butter, and oil frying in restaurant food may not be healthy. However, I see a shift like buying food from farmer's market[s] and eating at home. It is the mindset. I

worked in hospitality. It is time to change our habits to health alternatives. For example, when watching games on TV, one does not have to eat burgers, fruit could be an alternative. It will . . . change [the] mindset. Also during party[s], healthy food could be a good choice. Restaurants can serve child size portion[s] [of the] same items from adult's menu instead of serving unhealthy food items.

Parents and teachers can help community members to educate themselves on how to find healthy food options that are economically reasonable and involve them in promoting overall healthy development for children by reaching out to various organizations.

For example, at ProCamps Worldwide—the "Mariano Rivera baseball instruction and fun" program at the Sports Underdome in Mount Vernon, New York—boys and girls from grades 1–8 were able to join Major League Baseball player, Mariano Rivera, to get tips and instruction that highlight the finer points of the game of baseball. They also had the opportunity to learn fundamentals by experiencing various stations that specialize in teaching the major skills of baseball as each camper participated in games and skills contests.

This event was a wonderful experience for children as they were able to meet and learn from MLB player Mariano Rivera about the importance of instruction as well as the fundamentals of the sport, all while having fun and being active. Parents were appreciative of the event as it motivated their children to partake in physical exercise on weekends. The event was open to all children from grades 1–8, not just student athletes. Some parents expressed how pleased they were and said that the value of this experience really could not be measured in money—for them and their children, it was priceless. They appreciated the fact that their children were able to connect with their friends as well as meet new friends at the event. It is important for role models to educate young children about the value of living a healthy lifestyle. They have immense power in helping children understand how they are able to withstand the challenges they face while playing their sport. Athletes are able to maintain their "game-ready" status by eating healthy, resting, and practicing proper hygiene, as well as doing physical exercise. Parents and teachers have the opportunity to expand this awareness by working together to help promote the same ideas and goals for the overall healthy development for children.

Doctors have the knowledge and resources to help families learn about community programs that benefit children and improve their health. Focusing on the community is especially important for children since they generally have little or no control over their environment.

Parents and teachers can get involved in the community by planting or creating more community gardens, participating in farmers' markets and community-supported agriculture projects or sponsoring free sports and exercise classes for children.

Some programs like New York Junior Tennis & Learning are free for children. This group uses tennis as a tool to change lives. There are a variety of great educational programs in schools and communities throughout all five boroughs. One of the most popular programs is the Community Tennis Program that teaches children (aged 6 to 18) how to play tennis by providing free training and support.

STEPS is a community-based childhood obesity intervention program. It is a family-focused health improvement program for children with a BMI over the 85th percentile for their age. Admission to the program is through referral from a physician or school nurse and addresses healthier diet choices, physical activity, and counseling to support behavioral change. The program is led by a registered dietitian, licensed social worker, and exercise specialist who work with both the child and their parents.

Shape Up NYC is a wonderful fitness program for the entire family and it's free! Simply go to the website to choose from a variety of active classes. There is something for everyone from preschoolers to seniors, and all five boroughs are covered. A recent search turned up a free "Intensati" workout class that "fuses high energy aerobics, martial arts, dance, yoga, and strength conditioning."

The New York City Department of Parks & Recreation offers various programs. Swimming is one of the most useful athletic undertakings and NYC residents can take advantage of free water-based programs in every borough. Free classes range from aquatics exercise to competitive swim team programs. There is something for all ages and experience levels, from beginners to expert swimmers.

CityParks Kids or the City Parks Foundation is known for many of its cultural offerings, and also offers some of the best free sports programs around. The CityParks Golf program provides free golf lessons for kids aged 6 to 17 and the recently opened CityParks Junior Golf Center, a six-hole golf course, provides further free instruction. Other sports highlights include a tennis program, which provides free tennis lessons to kids aged 5 to 16, and a summer track and field program. These are excellent and free opportunities for children!

The Kids Food Festival is a weekend event focusing on educating families about making balanced food choices through fun and flavorful activities. The exciting and engaging programming of the Kids Food Festival helps to establish wholesome lifelong habits, while working to avert childhood obesity.

The mission of the festival is to aid in the transformation toward balanced eating habits through education and promotion of sensible food choices. They aim to reduce childhood obesity by generating a greater demand for wholesome and balanced food products through education, sampling, and exposure. They also aim to facilitate collaborations between families, communities, businesses, schools, and public and nonprofit organizations to help create a healthier food environment for kids.

New York City parents lead busy lives but still want to provide their kids with nutritious food options. Good thing delivery isn't just for adults! NYC has plenty to offer in the way of culinary delights sent directly to your door, including food-delivery services that specialize in healthy meals for kids. Whether you want vegan food for your baby or organic treats for your toddler, these delivery options will satisfy your kids' appetites with healthy options.

Petit Organics provides handmade organic and vegan baby food to families throughout Manhattan which is free of preservatives, artificial flavors and colors, added salts and sugars, and genetically engineered ingredients. The Petit Pack ($48) contains a three-day supply of baby food in nine four-ounce containers; order online, and choose between a preset variety pack or a create-your-own combination of different purees and blends, with ingredients such as apples, pears, oats, and cinnamon. You can pick up the food at any of Petit's five locations, or choose a delivery date and time. The food is prepared less than 24 hours before being delivered to your doorstep and arrives in cold packaging, but should be refrigerated immediately.

Little Green Gourmets produces a diverse selection of healthy snacks, lunches, and dinners for children. Using organic and local ingredients, the delivery service aims to help parents raise "smart eaters." By joining its e-mail list, you'll receive menus and selection forms each week. Order meals à la carte and have them delivered directly to your home, or order by subscription for delivery to participating schools.

Junior's Fresh provides handcrafted, farm-fresh food for the urban child. Junior's Fresh is committed to making tasty meals with seasonal ingredients from local farms. Eschewing synthetic fertilizers, pesticides, herbicides, artificial colors and flavors, fungicides, preservatives, and GMO seeds, meals are made 24 hours before delivery and are good for up to four days. Junior's Fresh makes food for babies four months and older that includes ingredients such as butternut squash, beets, and quinoa.

Shoogies NYC, located in Manhattan or Brooklyn, provides foods babies and toddlers can enjoy such as Shoogies' all-natural organic meals. Containing no preservatives and nothing artificial, the Shoogies menu includes purees with ingredients such as broccoli, cauliflower, and apple for babies five to ten months old, and meals such as hummus and pita or grilled cheese for children ten months and older.

Komi Organics delivers freshly made meals that include nutrients beneficial to your growing children, such as DHA, B12, and choline. Komi seeks to promote overall health and cognitive development through nutritious food choices. This service provides all-natural meals that are low in sodium and do not contain added sugars, preservatives, or additives.

Parents need to involve their children in sports. There are many recreational centers where parents can enroll their children in various activities. Watch for signs hung up on the street that advertise free recreational activities that are scheduled weekly at dance studios, community parks, camps, and fitness centers.

In New York, some dance studios that children can attend in the community are: Just For Kicks School of Dance, Leggz Dance Studio, Ballet of Long Island, Broadway Dance Academy, JAM For Children, and so many more. All dance studios are privately owned and offer endless opportunities for physical movement. Other recreational programs that are offered in the community are: The JCC, Sportset Gym, and ROK Fitness.

These gym-related environments offer classes for children. For example, Sportset Gym, located in Rockville Center, New York, offers children yoga class as well as karate and fitness classes. Teachers in this program give children the opportunity to see what they can really do.

Parents and teachers can involve the community in promoting overall healthy development for children in numerous ways. Health issues are arising so quickly because of the lifestyle that humans live. The degree of access we have to fast-food chains, transportation services, and electronics is a lot. All of these factors contribute to reasons why children are unhealthy and possibly struggling from obesity. It cannot be stressed enough that families, teachers, and communities need to encourage children to become more active in their daily lives.

In spring, summer, and fall, parents should be taking their children outdoors for walks and runs. Teachers should be open to taking their students outside for a learning activity or field trip. The outdoor lesson can consist of students hopping, skipping, jumping, twirling, etc. All lesson plans should involve some type of physical activity. This will decrease the statistics of obesity and increase children's overall development of health.

A few fast-food chains have offered more healthy options lately. Subway and Wendy's are offering salads, and other restaurants are offering low-fat dressing and mayonnaise. There are also a few healthy food chains, such as Just Salad, Chipotle, and Whole Foods. These restaurants provide healthier, more natural food that is easily accessible.

Overall, more restaurants need to get on board with helping community health as a whole. They can start by using organic ingredients and offering healthier menu options for the consumer. It is important as a community that we advertise healthy restaurants.

Parents can request that local food businesses as well as fast-food restaurants have nutrition facts readily available for families to look through so they can make healthy, informed decisions when they are eating out. Parents and teachers can scout out all-natural and organic restaurants and stores and request that they deliver menus throughout the neighborhood so that families will have healthier options. Providing children and their parents with the skills to search for these types of places on the Internet or on their smartphones will help them in their journey to a healthier lifestyle as well.

Physical and cultural activities can also take place at events where families within the community share different foods, music, and sports with each other. Children can feel a sense of belonging, be physically active, improve their social-emotional skills, and learn about cultures that are different than their own when people get together.

The accessibility of recreational facilities, food stores that offer healthy and affordable choices, and available physical activity in a community all influence children's health values and habits. People who live in a community that has many fast-food places are more likely to become obese, but a person living in a community with access to local food stores is more likely to choose healthier life-style habits.

Poorer neighborhoods have three times fewer supermarkets than wealthier neighborhoods but contain more fast-food restaurants and convenient stores, constraining residents' ability to access healthy food locally. A higher density of fast-food restaurants, along with concentrated media marketing, promotes unhealthy food choices and hinders good nutrition.

Strategies to build a partnership among the home environment, schools, and organizations across the community can encourage the expansion of health-care facilities to serve as better models of healthy lifestyles. Communities can collaborate to raise money for parks and recreational facilities so that families can go to and engage in physical activities that are enjoyed by parents and their children together.

The importance of community on child health and development is crucial. One is incomplete without the other. Children and the community prosper from a successful collaboration. "Healthy children are raised by people and communities." Communities play a large role in how children develop; they can offer resources such as parks, school programs, and childcare facilities. Families make a community, therefore members in the community should have an understanding that working together is beneficial for all.

The following guideline helps families in New York understand the importance of the food we choose and is a helpful resource on how to make the right selections. "The U.S. Department of Health and Human Services (HHS) is committed to making the information from the Dietary Guidelines and Physical Activity Guidelines accessible to the majority of the U.S. adult population."

"Eat Healthy, Be Active" community workshops promote knowledge as power to making better choices. They encourage families to make small changes in the pursuit of a lifelong healthy lifestyle. Many families have issues understanding why the local fast-food options are the wrong options for their children.

Being role models for your children will help guide them to maintain a balanced and healthy life. Although we are all busy and time is limited, making home-cooked meals is crucial to improving the health of our families. It is even possible to make the child's favorite food meal at home as a healthy alternative. Being sure to incorporate nutritious food full of proteins and whole grains will keep children energized and full longer and help them to avoid poor choices (Batra & Media, 2012).

In order for the community to get involved in promoting healthy development for children, government policy makers, health professionals, and community residents must work in unison toward this cause. An example of policy makers working together for change is the NYC Community Parks Initiative program, which works directly with New Yorkers to transform the neighborhoods with the greatest needs for parks. The Community Parks Initiative offers immediate physical improvement and enhanced public programming at sites across the city.

Law makers contribute to the health and wellness of children as well. The state government also plays a crucial role in providing children with a community that promotes healthy development. "Every child deserves a bright, green space right in their neighborhoods" (Foderaro, 2015). The New York State Department of Health has a focus area of reducing obesity in children by creating community environments that promote and support healthy food and beverage choices and physical activity (New York State Prevention Agenda 2013–2018: Priorities, Focus Areas, Goals and Objectives, 2015).

One way the New York state government promotes healthy food options to the community is by providing NYC green carts, which are mobile food carts that offer fresh produce in New York City neighborhoods with limited access to healthy foods. Fruits and vegetables are the only things sold on green carts.

In order to prevent the obesity epidemic, it is paramount for families, schools, and communities to collaborate with one another in a multitude of ways. A school that promotes health and nutrition should also have some type of rapport with local markets and shops that exemplify healthy nutrition. This type of openness to collaborate will create healthy opportunities for children.

For example, the use of promotions creates money-saving and nutritious shopping opportunities for parents and healthy lifestyle choices for the child. Similarly, schools can organize trips to strawberry- or apple-picking fields. Having and utilizing these types of relationships among community, families, and schools gives children experiences in enriching environments. Engaging students in such activities not only stimulates a nutritious diet to fight the obesity epidemic, it also educates students on the importance of understanding nature and its produce.

Even more importantly, it provides the children with a multisensory experience and an experience in the community which promotes a child's sense of belonging in their neighborhood. Schools can then further take advantage of such collaborative relationships by organizing class trips to local markets and community health centers.

Parents should follow up by revisiting these places with their child in order to make these healthy resources that the child has familiarity with and can learn to enjoy in an independent manner. Schools should also emphasize communicating valuable nutrition tips and materials to parents. These techniques and materials should preferably be used in the classroom in order to create a family-like school.

Growing their own fruits and vegetables can help strengthen children's habits of eating healthy foods. Community gardening is one of the strategies that can prevent obesity among children. Community gardens can be used to provide children proper nutrition and healthy eating. Participating in a community garden also provides family time together.

According to a study of a community garden–based obesity prevention program among low-income families, "By the end of their participation in the program, 17% of obese or overweight children had improved their BMI classification and 100% of the children with a BMI classification of normal had maintained that BMI. According to the parental reports, there was an increase of 146% in the availability of fruits and vegetables and an increase in the consumption of fruits (28%) and vegetables (33%) among children of families participating in the program" (Castro, Samuels, & Harmon, 2013).

At school, there are several strategies that will help prevent childhood obesity. Putting refrigerators in classroom may encourage students to bring their own lunch/snacks from home. Parents can pack healthy foods instead of children having school-provided lunch or other foods that are less likely to contain healthy ingredients.

Removing vending machines with unhealthy foods and drinks or replacing these items with healthy snacks is another strategy. "A prospective study involving middle-school students over the course of 2 academic years showed that the risk of becoming obese increased by 60% for every additional serving of sugar-sweetened beverages per day" (Brownell, 2009).

Children could develop healthy active behaviors. Restaurants can get involved in promoting healthy development of the children. There is a program called Kids LiveWell, launched by the National Restaurant Association, which showcases restaurants that offer healthful menu options for children.

The program is participated in by a lot of restaurants including well-known chain restaurants such as Au Bon Pain, Burger King, Denny's, Friendly's, IHOP, Outback Steakhouse, and Sizzler, etc. Restaurants participating in the Kids LiveWell program offer at least one full children's menu item that is 600 calories or less, contains fruits, vegetables, and limits sodium, fats, and sugar. Also offered is at least one other individual item that has 200 calories or less.

According to a student, "Of the children who reported ordering kids' meals, more than half said that they would be somewhat or very likely to order a kid's meal that came with vegetables (56.2% of tweens: 54.8% of teens) or fruits (78.9% of tweens; 73% of teens)" (Anzman-Frasca et al., 2014).

As one of community members, I interviewed a restaurant owner. She said that she has her own grandsons and daughter eating at the restaurant. She was very concerned about foods that they eat, which motivated her to provide food made with healthy ingredients. The first thing she does when she makes food is to try to eliminate any MSG. She hasn't researched or studied whether MSG affects people's health, but knowing that it is bad for health she stopped using it.

The other thing she tries to do is provide and use more vegetables. Since she owns a buffet-style restaurant, she has increased the number of foods that have more vegetables. She created a greater variety of salads among the food choices. She also provides 100 percent juice or tea free to her young customers so they can avoid drinking sugar-sweetened beverages or sodas.

It was probably a hard decision to use higher-priced ingredients or to think about other people's health as a person who wants to make a profit, but it sets a good example. If more community members like her would take such initiatives, children would naturally learn how to stay healthy and develop healthy behaviors.

A community can promote the healthy development of children by building gym or fitness centers that offer special programs or offer discount memberships for children. Some schools advertise free Taekwondo (Korean martial arts) classes for their students. Taekwondo requires great physical movement, which can help overweight students and help promote more physical activity.

There are community organizations, such as the YMCA, which offer programs that children can enjoy with their families. They have programs like "Family Time" where families participate in a variety of fun activities including pool games, crafts, family fitness, camping, hiking, and swimming that will provide an environment to build bonds through shared experiences.

A study used a method called "Healthy Schools," where students had access to a gymnasium, playground, sports field, and rooms for table and board games. The study followed a control group and an intervention group. It found that students taking part in the "Healthy Schools" program were taking more steps on a daily basis, and that "the proportions of obese and overweight participants declined." It also found that students in the intervention group had more physical activity on weekends and more leisure time than those not involved in the intervention (Sigmund, Ansari, & Sigmundova, 2012).

Research performed by the CDC (2016), showed that the health of students is directly linked to academic success. Students need adequate nutrition, proper rest, and enough physical activity to demonstrate optimum academic performance. The website suggested nine guidelines in promoting healthy eating and physical activity in schools:

1. Use a coordinated approach to develop, implement, and evaluate healthy eating and physical activity policy and practices.
2. Establish school environments that support healthy eating and physical activity.
3. Provide a quality school meal program and ensure that students have only appealing, healthy food and beverage choices offered outside of the school meal program.
4. Implement a comprehensive physical activity program with quality physical education as the cornerstone.
5. Implement health education that provides students with the knowledge, attitudes, skills and experiences needed for lifelong healthy eating and physical activity.
6. Provide students with health, mental health, and social services to address healthy eating, physical activity, and related chronic disease prevention.
7. Partner with families and community members in the development and implementation of healthy eating and physical activity policies, practices, and programs.
8. Provide a school employee wellness program that includes healthy eating and physical activity services for all school staff members.
9. Employ qualified persons, and provide professional development opportunities for physical education, health education, and nutrition services, and health, mental health, and social services staff members, as well as staff members who supervise recess, cafeteria time, and out-of-school-time programs.

10. Provide staff members who supervise recess, cafeteria time, and out of school time programs.

(https://cdc.gov/healthyschools/npao/strategies)

Whether you are teaching early childhood, elementary, middle, or high school, there are ways that you can incorporate physical fitness and health into the curriculum. As stated earlier, providing students with lists of free events can help encourage them to get involved in their community and exercise. Arranging class trips to places like the YMCA, or even to supermarkets like Shop Rite, encourages students to think about the choices they are making when it comes to health and nutrition.

Assigning research topics to older students about health-related topics is also a good way to start an open conversation in the classroom in English, science, health and even social studies classes. Students can present group projects on health-related topics. If you are teaching physical education, you can even assign a group project where students have to design a five-minute exercise routine and teach it to the class.

Some schools have even devoted an entire month to promoting healthy habits, where students explore different foods, activities, and learn about living a healthy lifestyle. Assigning an exercise log to students can also help them self-assess just how much exercise they are getting on a daily basis, and may help motivate them to become more active.

The school functions as a microcommunity and administration can utilize various community programs to help foster healthy practices within their school. If a school creates a community within their building where health and wellness is valued, it can help the entire student body become healthier and more active.

This can be accomplished by creating more after-school activities that encourage physical movement. Schools can have one day a week where they offer an after-school fitness class, or they can create a sports team, which also fosters a sense of teamwork, and can help students develop a sense of belonging to build higher self-esteem.

Studies also show that students focus better when they are allowed to be physically active in the classroom, and that giving students an "exercise break" actually helps students become more focused during the school day. This can be accomplished by taking five minutes in between subjects to have students stretch and do something as simple as jumping jacks or running in place. It also helps break the monotony between subjects and in transitioning between activities.

The school administration can reach out to community board members and invite them to speak at the school. They can discuss activities that are going on in the community, and offer students extra credit for attending the events and writing a small review of it.

The school can hold a health fair where projects created by the students that focus on health and wellness are displayed. Local businesses dealing with health and wellness can be invited to set up booths in the auditorium where they can promote their enterprises. A dance festival is a great way to get students active, and can also help students explore other cultures and heritages. School-wide walks for charity are also a great way to get students moving. They also help foster a strong school identity, while giving back to the community, and to those less fortunate.

Schools need to be aware that while they are encouraging healthy habits, they also want to encourage tolerance and acceptance. The goal should be health, not fitting into a socially mandated body stereotype. Schools should make sure that all staff are on the same page when discussing body and weight issues, and parents should be made aware that these topics are going to be discussed so that they can continue the discussion at home. A well-designed program will foster feelings of inclusion, support, and encouragement.

Parents, medical professionals, educators, and our legislative officials need to form a new team to fight obesity. The long-term consequences of childhood obesity are real, but with some lifestyle changes, they can be avoided. It's up to us, as a community, to take action, to encourage and support our children to make better choices, and to live a healthier lifestyle.

It is important that home, school, and community work together to prevent the spread of the obesity epidemic. Some of the strategies are communities and neighborhoods that limit fast food restaurants in the area, improving restaurant menu offerings for children, and increasing the availability of farmers markets and community gardens.

Further strategies to encourage physical activity include establishing parks, playgrounds, bike paths, and routes for walking or bicycling to school, as well as developing programs to encourage walking and bicycling to school. To increase physical activity, children can walk to school instead of taking a school bus or parents drive to school. A study by Mori et al. (2012) discusses a program in Japan where "about 98.3% of children walk or cycle to school and this program was implemented for many decades. This program has been associated with increased activity among the school-going children" and has led to a lower prevalence of obesity among the teenagers in the country.

MARKETING TO CHILDREN AND YOUTH

Food corporations have significantly contributed to the obesity epidemic. Their marketing strategies have played a decisive role in the development of this health crisis, nationally and internationally. The food industry targets children and youth to market their products. Each year over $1.6 billion is spent to market products to young people. *BioMed Central* found that for every 10 percent increase in food advertising in urban neighborhoods, the odds of high obesity levels increased significantly.

Further, in 2009, the fast-food industry spent over $4.2 billion on TV, radio, magazine, and outdoor advertising, and other forms of media. The fast-food industry, with its growing popularity, focuses on children and exists wherever they are, following them into their homes or schools via television, Internet, or cell phones, etc.

Focusing on children at an early age and marketing directly to them affects their food choices, food preferences, and eating habits. Each day, children face the enticing advertisements of unhealthy food. In 2012, fast-food restaurants spent $4.6 billion in total advertising, an 8 percent increase over 2009. For context, the biggest advertiser, McDonald's, spent 2.7 times as much to advertise its products as all fruit, vegetable, bottled water, and milk advertisers combined.

Companies like McDonald's target younger demographics, contributing to high obesity rates today. The McDonald's Corporation focuses on children so they are at places where children are. They are prominently represented in video games, on book jackets, and even in theme parks. Children may receive free toys with their "Happy Meals" or watch celebrities and movie characters endorse products. By connecting food products to pop culture, corporations generate enthusiasm among their young targets, who then influence their parents' purchasing choices.

A 2010 study by the Yale University Rudd Center for Food Policy and Obesity (Folkvord et al., 2015) found that 40 percent of parents reported that their child asked to eat at McDonald's at least once a week. If the children are pleading to eat at McDonald's once a week, then it is definitely because these fast-food restaurants are enticing the children with fatty foods and popular toys.

McDonald's display advertisements for "Happy Meals" increased 63 percent to 31 million advertisements monthly. Three-quarters of the ads appeared on kids' websites, such as nick.com, roblox.com, and cartoonnetwork.com. These are very popular among children and also children talk to their friends at school who watch these shows. Therefore, the advertisements during these popular shows catch young children's attention right away and with repeated advertisements in different shows, children tend to believe in what they see.

Often it is seen that children also memorize advertisements. Therefore, most fast-food restaurants find success in reaching children and so they step up advertising to children. These fast-food restaurants target children as young as preschoolers. Preschoolers' exposure to TV advertising did not change at all, or perhaps increased. In 2012, preschoolers saw 1,023 fast-food advertisements—2.8 per day. Three-fifths of fast-food restaurants increased TV advertising to older children.

Research has found a strong relationship between an increase in advertising for nonnutritious foods and the rates of childhood obesity. On an average, children between the ages of two and seventeen watch twelve to twenty-one television commercials for food products daily (McManus, 2016). There are many compelling advertisements aimed at both children and their parents.

Popular cartoon characters or celebrities promote sugary foods as "a great source of whole grains." The truth about these sugary foods, especially cereals, is not unveiled. Children, after viewing those advertisements, use "pester power" and often plead with and beg their parents to buy those unhealthy products until their parents finally give in. Parents on the other hand also lack knowledge and become prey to the deception of these advertisements.

Today's children, from ages eight to eighteen years old, consume multiple types of media, sometimes simultaneously. They spend more time, approximately 44.5 hours per week, in front of computer, television, and game screens than on any other activity in their lives. Research has found strong relationships between the increase in advertising for nonnutritious foods and rates of child-hood obesity; most children under age six cannot distinguish between programming and advertising, and children under age eight do not understand the persuasive intent of advertising.

Advertising directed at children this young is by its very nature exploitative. Children at this age are vulnerable and absorb everything they see or hear like sponges. They also have a remarkable ability to recall content from the advertisements to which they have been exposed. On television, advertisements occur with as little as a single commercial exposure or are strengthened with repeated exposures. Exposure to unhealthy food advertisements affects children's product purchase requests and these requests influence parents' purchasing decisions.

Research has demonstrated the strong effect of marketing about the type and quantity of food that people eat. In one research study (Harris et al., 2009), elementary school children watched a cartoon that contained either a food-related or a non-food-related advertisement. The children who watched the food advertisement consumed 45 percent more of the snack they were given afterward. This study indicated that children believed what they saw and it creates a lasting impression.

A study (Folkvord et al., 2015) of ninety-two children examined the effect of food-related or non-food-related content in a video game on eating habits. It was found that the kids exposed to food advertisements within the game chose snacks with greater caloric density and ate significantly more. American children and youth expose themselves to excessive amounts of television. Parents often use television as a babysitter. From another study, conducted by the Kaiser Family Foundation (2006), it was found that 79 percent of children reported one hour or more of daily television exposure.

Subtle messages about food, often specifically designed to trigger the body's hunger response, have become an integral part of the typical television viewing experience. A review of advertising techniques done by Yale Rudd (Folkvord et al., 2015), found that fast-food commercials directly aimed at children have increased by 28 percent and adolescents today see 40 percent more restaurant advertisements than in 2002. This increase contributes significantly to the obesity epidemic because the malleable and delicate minds of children make them easy prey for advertisements.

TELEVISION ADVERTISEMENTS CONTRIBUTE TO CHILDHOOD OBESITY

Food advertisements on television make up 50 percent of all the advertisement time on children's shows. These advertisements are almost completely dominated by unhealthy food products (34 percent for candy and snacks, 28 percent for cereal, 10 percent for fast food, 4 percent for dairy products, 1 percent for fruit juices, and 0 percent for fruits or vegetables). Therefore, the above data indicated that children are rarely exposed to public service announcements or advertising for healthier foods (Kaiser Family Foundation, 2007).

Obesity in children increases the more hours they watch television. Children's exposure to TV ads for unhealthy food products (that is, high-calorie, low-nutrient snacks, fast foods, and sweetened drinks) are a significant risk factor for obesity. In very young children, research has found that for every one-hour increase in TV viewing per day, there are higher intakes of sugar-sweetened beverages, fast food, red and processed meat, and overall calories (48.7 kcal/day).

Excess weight can be gained by the addition of only 150 calories a day. Other research has found that children who watch more than three hours of television a day are 50 percent more likely to be obese than children who watch fewer than two hours. This is alarming to note that watching TV for two hours or three hours can make such a huge difference with regard to obesity.

Food and beverage advertising targeted at children influences their product preferences, requests, and diets. The food and beverage industry has resolved to self-regulate its marketing to children, but this has not resulted in significant improvement in the marketing of healthier foods (such as fruits, vegetables, whole grains, low-fat or nonfat milk or dairy products, lean meats, poultry, fish and beans) to children. Almost three out of every four foods advertised to children falls into the unhealthy categories that contribute to the obesity epidemic. Children's level of exposure to these ads by age can be found in the table below.

Per the table, it is clearly seen that children between the ages of eight and twelve are receiving the highest rates of ad exposure. They are entering a critical stage of development where they are establishing food habits, making more of their own food choices, and have their own money to spend on the types of food they enjoy.

MARKETING OF FOOD ONLINE TO CHILDREN

Marketing of food to children on the Internet is even more complex since the boundaries between content and pure advertising are often less clear than on television. Only a minority of advertisers include reminders distinguishing content from pure advertising. One study (Kaiser Family Foundation, 2004) has shown that children find it harder to recognize advertisements on websites than they do on television; six-year-olds only recognized a quarter of the advertisements, eight-year-olds recognized half of the advertisements, and

Table 6.1. Children's Exposure Levels to TV Ads for Unhealthy Foods

Ages	Ads per day	Hours per year	Ads per year	Exposure to PSAs
2–7	12	29:31	4,427	1 every 2–3 days
8–12	21	50:48	7,609	1 every 2–3 days
13–17	17	40:50	6,098	< 1 every week

ten- and twelve-year-olds recognized about three-quarters of the advertisements.

The majority of food brands advertised to children on TV are also promoted on the Internet and often include online games which are heavily branded, known as "advergames." Advergames can provide a more highly involving and entertaining brand experience than what is possible with conventional media.

Websites also contain other brand-related content such as television commercials, promotions, viral marketing, and website membership opportunities. Viral marketing is used to encourage children to talk to one another about a brand's website by emailing friends in the form of an e-greeting or invitation and inviting them to visit the site. Marketers also often provide brand-related items that can be downloaded or printed and saved, for example, brand-related screensavers and wallpapers.

The continual branding through these sites reinforces and amplifies the product message to children, and children have a remarkable ability to recall content from advertisements to which they are exposed.

IN-SCHOOL ADVERTISING

There is also a creeping commercialism finding its way into America's schools. Children spend a considerable amount of their time in school settings, where compulsory attendance makes it difficult to avoid exposure to commercial content. Commercial content delivered in schools may be assumed to have the tacit endorsement of respected teachers and school officials, thereby enhancing the effectiveness of the advertising. Food and beverage advertising exists in 70 percent of elementary and middle schools and in 90 percent of high schools. Companies integrate themselves into students' social lives. Nearly half of US middle and high schools allow advertising of less healthy food. They claim advertisement space in cafeterias, sponsor school dances, and even fund athletic programs.

Advertising and marketing in schools takes several forms, including direct and indirect advertising. Direct advertising in school classrooms is by advertiser-sponsored video or audio programming. Indirect advertising is by corporate-sponsored educational materials. Further, there are product sales contracts with soda and snack-food companies.

Advertisements are now appearing on school buses, in gymnasiums, on book covers, and even in bathroom stalls. School advertising also appears under the guise of educational TV. For instance, Channel One, which is available in 12,000 schools, provides programming consisting of 10 minutes of current events and 2 minutes of commercials. Advertisers pay $200,000 for advertising time and the opportunity to target 40 percent of the nation's teenagers for 30 seconds (Wartella and Jennings, 2001). It is quite shocking to discover how much money advertisers pay to reach the target audience.

Fast-food restaurants should stop marketing directly to children and teens to encourage consumption of unhealthy fast food. They can limit advertising on children's TV networks and third-party kids' websites to healthy kids' meals only.

It is time to stop unfair marketing targeted at children, including advertisements that focus on promotions, not food, mobile advergame apps, and online ads that link to advergame sites. They should ensure that preschoolers are not exposed to fast-food advertising, especially advertising on Spanish-language TV. They should stop targeting older children as young as age twelve with marketing for unhealthy fast food that can damage their health. We need to establish age limits on fast-food marketing to youth via social media and mobile devices that takes unfair advantage of their susceptibility to peer influence and impulsive actions.

A recent study (Dickey, 2015) found that fast-food commercials featuring toy giveaways led children to ask their parents to take them to the restaurants. And the more the children saw the fast-food commercials, the more frequently they ate fast food. The study, performed by researchers from Dartmouth's Geisel School of Medicine, focused on the advertising of Burger King and McDonald's, the two major fast-food brands on ad-supported children's networks such as Nickelodeon and Cartoon Network.

Nearly 70 percent of the food ads during *SpongeBob Square-Pants*, *Teenage Mutant Ninja Turtles*, *The Fairly Odd Parents*, *iCarly*, and other popular children's shows on the Nickelodeon network are for junk foods, according to the Center for Science in the Public Interest (CSPI).

CSPI researchers catalogued the food advertising on 28 hours of Nickelodeon programming in October 2012 and found eighty-eight advertisements for foods. Of those, 69 percent were for foods of poor nutritional quality. The most common products marketed to kids were sugary cereals, candy, yogurt with added sugars, fast-food and other restaurants, and snacks (cspinet.org, 2016).

Nevertheless, "Nickelodeon congratulates itself for running the occasional public service announcement promoting physical activity," said CSPI nutrition policy director Margo G. Wootan. "But for each of those messages, it's running 30 advertisements for junk food. Nickelodeon is clearly doing far more harm than good when it comes to the health of America's young people." Junk food is making kids overweight and contributing to the onset of type 2 diabetes and other health problems.

CASE STUDY: A RESTAURANT'S FOOD QUALITY

While homemade food is ideal, with busy schedules, every now and then families take a break to dine at restaurants. Hence, the author focused on a research study on preventing obesity and finding out the quality of nutrition in the food served in restaurants. In a specific restaurant in the author's community, the customers were requested to complete a survey questionnaire about the food quality.

The researcher also communicated with the customers to see how they felt about the food they were being served. Further, the researcher communicated with the cook to receive his input on the food he makes. The results yielded that the customers were quite satisfied with the quality of food in the restaurant.

A lot of chain restaurants are labeling menus to provide consumers with calorie counts and other information about standard menu items. Evidence about the impact of menu labeling on customers' purchase intentions as well as on actual purchases and their corresponding calories is rapidly growing.

This research review summarizes new information from Healthy Eating Research. Key findings show that there is a high degree of public support for providing nutrition information during purchase, and menu labeling in restaurants increases consumers' awareness of nutritional information. It also finds that menu labeling may impact some customers and types of menu items more than others, and menu labeling may have a positive influence on the nutritional content of menu items and restaurant environments, for example, reduction in the promotion of less healthy foods (Research Review, Robert Wood Johnson Foundation, 2013).

From the Scientific Blogging article, "On Surveys, Customers Prefer Restaurants That Offer Health Food" (2014), it was found that, generally, when people go out to restaurants, they don't care about eating healthy. Fast-food restaurants have been convinced to spend tens of millions of dollars marketing healthy choices for kids, like apples, however, they claim that they are basically invisible to children.

People don't want to overpay for the same food they will get at home and they don't care about labels. But when they fill out surveys they will claim to care about labels, which is not the same thing. When it comes to food, behavior and claims are often radically different. However, the study claimed that the customers are more likely to frequent restaurants that provide both healthful foods and nutrition information.

The results from the study suggest that when a restaurant presented nutrition information and served healthful food options, survey participants were significantly more likely to perceive that the restaurant was socially responsible, regardless of their level of health-consciousness. These results also indicated that highly health-conscious people are more sensitive to healthy foods at restaurants than less health-conscious people, regardless of whether or not nutrition information is provided.

Another study by Platkin et al. (2014) examined the effect of menu labeling with calorie information and exercise equivalents on food selection. They stated that better techniques are needed to help consumers in restaurants make lower-calorie food choices. The results yielded that menu labeling alone may be insufficient to reduce consumption of calories.

In this study, customers were quite satisfied with the food quality they get in the restaurant. Customers preferred healthy choices of food as they are concerned with the type of food they eat. However, only 50 percent said that they would like to get information about the ingredients of the food and how it is cooked, and the other 50 percent said that they do not want such information. In this particular restaurant where the study was done, the cook stated that less oil is now used in food per customers' requests, and olive oil is used in salads.

However, this is not the case with every restaurant. Other restaurants use a lot of oil in the some dishes. Customers need to be aware of the food quality they get. If customers are proactive, the problem of weight issues could be reduced.

Although there are some positive trends in food marketing to teens, fast-food restaurants continue to target them with TV and Internet ads for primarily unhealthy products. It is in the hands of adults and consumers to control their weight and maintain their health. Television advertisements viewed by teens did not change, but average calories per advertisements viewed declined by 16 percent. However, teens were more likely to see more television advertisements for Taco Bell, Sonic, and Starbucks when compared with adults. It is good news that displays of advertisements on youth websites declined by more than half, from 470 million monthly advertisements views per month in 2009 to 210 million in 2012. However, KFC, Subway, and Starbucks more than doubled display advertising on youth websites (Yale Rudd Center, 2013).

The most alarming news is that fast-food marketing via mobile devices and social media popular with teens has grown exponentially. Six billion fast-food advertisements appeared on Facebook— 19 percent of all fast-food display advertising—including more than half of Dunkin' Donuts' and Wendy's advertisements. Further, smartphone apps offer interactive features such as order functions and special offers. These apps on smartphones are becoming very popular among teenagers.

Alarmingly, fast-food restaurants continue to target African American and Hispanic youth. Records indicate that these youth are more likely than others to visit one-third or more of all fast-food websites. Moreover, African American and Hispanic youth face a higher risk for obesity and related diseases. Fast-food advertising spending on Spanish-language television increased by 8 percent. However, KFC and Burger King increased their spending by 35 to 41 percent while reducing English-language advertising.

Over the last three years, there have been some improvements in the nutritional quality of fast food and in companies' marketing practices. However, the pace of improvement is slow and unlikely to reduce young people's overconsumption of high-calorie, nutritionally poor fast food.

Fast-food restaurants should do more to improve the nutritional quality of kids' meals and regular menu items. They can apply industry standards for healthy kids' meals to the majority of kids' meal combinations available for purchase, not a mere 3 percent. They should automatically provide healthy sides and beverages as the default kids' meals. They could increase the proportion of lower-calorie, healthier items on their menus and make them available at a reasonable price.

Without policy makers' intervention and increased government regulation of food advertising and a shift in public views on all of this marketing, the obesity epidemic will continue to expand. Under the Obama administration, the White House and the Department of Agriculture laid out new restrictions to limit advertisements for unhealthy foods on school grounds.

However, restrictions can be hard to implement because food companies are wealthy, well-connected, and accustomed to self-regulation. They argue that the right to free speech extends to corporations, which justifies their right to advertise free from governmental oversight. The attempt to regulate school-based advertisements, although it springs from good intentions, lacks the power to spur real progress.

Departments of education in different states need to incorporate nutrition courses into their curricula, mixing the importance of vegetables and the dangers of advertising into classes that will create savvy consumers. The best course of action lies in public education and the regulation of fast-food and advertising corporations. Food companies are making America's children obese, so we as a nation must begin to control it immediately.

RECOMMENDATIONS FOR PARENTS

It is recommended that parents encourage active, healthy lifestyles for children and adolescents, to include moderate television viewing, regular family mealtimes, and regular exercise. Parents must limit excessive time spent watching TV, video, gaming, or surfing the web. It is strongly recommended that parents monitor the media that children consume, particularly if they are under age eight.

Further, encourage healthy eating habits (that is, greater consumption of fruits, vegetables, whole grains, low-fat or nonfat milk or dairy products, lean meats, poultry, fish, and beans) and promote physical activity. Try dining with your kids and take pleasure in your mealtimes together. Lead by example by eating healthy foods and engaging in physical activity yourself. Remember you can have the greatest influence on your children's health.

TV time could also be family time when as a family you'll probably see four or five ads for fast food on TV. Since kids younger than eight will believe almost anything advertisements tell them, that is the time when parents can explain to children that what they see in the advertisements may not be healthy for them. Parents can teach children to make good choices in the face of fast-food advertisements. Mainly, try not to get distracted.

Also the next time you see a fast-food commercial, time how long it takes before you get information about the food itself. Sometimes words like "natural," "organic," and "fresh" sound great, but you can't always take them at face value. A popular catchphrase doesn't make a food a healthy choice.

It is most important that parents and children learn about calorie counts. If you're a boy aged 13–18, you need between 2,200 and 3,200 calories a day. Girls the same age need fewer than that, around 1,800–2,400 calories a day. Parents need to teach children to say "no" to soda because it offers zero nutrition; it's just a way to deliver sugar and, in many cases, caffeine. You must learn to demand better. The more that teenagers stand up and argue back and really try to fight for their rights to be taken seriously as a consumer group that actually cares about health, the more companies will listen.

Lastly, be careful and try to "unfollow" your fast food. Any time you "like" or follow a fast-food chain on social media to get deals, or enter your email for a contest, you're handing marketers an all-access pass to your info—and to your attention.

DISCUSSION QUESTIONS

1. What are some of the ways parents can get involved in the community in promoting overall healthy development for children?
2. What are some of the ways teachers can help parents get involved in the community in promoting overall healthy development for children?
3. Make a list of all the dance and sports programs in your community.
4. Make a list of the types of food and stores that exist in your community.
5. Make a list of the types of restaurants that exist in your community. Get the menus and evaluate if the food served is healthy or unhealthy.
6. Help children make up a restaurant menu of all the types of food items children would like to see being served and list the prices.
7. How can your community help prevent obesity?

REFERENCES

Batra, S., and D. Media. 2012. How to keep kids away from fast food. Retrieved from http://healthyeating.sfgate.com/keep-kids-away-fast-food-3441.html.

Folkvord, F., D. J. Anschutz, R. W. Wiers,and M. Buijzen, M. 2015. The role of attentional bias in the effect of food advertising on actual food intake among children. *Appetite* 84: 251–58.

Goodwin, J. 2011. Obese kids may face social, emotional woes. *Daily Health News* (September 21). https://www.rxshop.md/news/9637/.

Harris, J. L., J. A. Bargh, and K. D. Brownell. 2009. Priming effects of television food advertising on eating behavior. *Health Psychology* 28 (4) (July): 404–13.

Kaiser Family Foundation. 2004. The role of media in childhood obesity: Issue brief. Retrieved from http://kff.org/other/issue-brief/the-role-of-media-in-childhood-obesity/.

———. 2006. It's child's play: Advergaming and the online marketing of food to children—Report. Retrieved from http://www.kff.org/entmedia/upload/7536.pdf.

———. 2007. Food for thought: Television food advertising to children in the United States. Retrieved from http://kff.org/other/food-for-thought-television-food-advertising-to/.

McManus, K. 2016. The impact of food advertising on childhood obesity. Retrieved from http://prowellness.vmhost.psu.edu/impact-food-advertising-childhood-obesity.

Montgomery, K., and J. Chester. 2011. Digital food marketing to children and adolescents. Retrieved from http://www.changelabsolutions.org/sites/default/files/DigitalMarketingReport_FINAL_web_20111017-rebrand.pdf.

Montgomery, M. 2016. Treating autism naturally plus strategies for prevention. *Natural Awakenings*, Long Island Edition.

Mori, N., F. Armada, and D. Willcox. 2012. Walking to school in Japan and childhood obesity prevention: New lessons from an old policy. *American Journal of Public Health* 102 (11) (September): 2068–73.

New York State Department of Health. 2015. New York State prevention agenda 2013–2018: Priorities, focus areas, goals and objectives, 1/25/2013 (revised March 16, 2015). Retrieved from https://www.health.ny.gov/prevention/prevention_agenda/2013-2017/tracking_indicators.htm.

Platkin, C., M.-C. Yeh, K. Hirsch, E. Wiewel, C. Lin, H. Tung, and V. H. Castellanos. 2014. The effect of menu labeling with calories and exercise equivalents on food selection and c consumption. Retrieved from https://bmcobes.biomedcentral.com/articles/10.1186/s40608-014-0021-5.

Robert Wood Johnson Foundation. 2013. Impact of menu labeling on customer behavior: A 2008–2012 update. *Healthy Eating Research (Research Review): Building evidence to prevent childhood obesity* (June): 1–23. Retrieved from http://healthyeatingresearch.org/wp-content/uploads/2013/12/HER-RR-Menu-Labeling-FINAL-6-2013.pdf.

Scientific Blogging News Staff. 2014. On surveys, customers prefer restaurants that offer health food. *Science 2.0* (April 1). Retrieved from http://www.science20.com/news_articles/on_surveys_customers_prefer_restaurants_that_offer_health_food-133109.

Sigmund, E., W. E. Ansari,, and D. Sigmundova. 2012. Does school-based physical activity decrease overweight and obesity in children aged 6–9 years? A
two-year nonrandomized longitudinal intervention study in the Czech Repub-
lic. *Biomedcentral*. Retrieved from https://bmcpublichealth.biomedcentral.
com/articles/10.1186/1471-2458-12-570.

The Rudd Center for Food Policy and Obesity. 2010. Retrieved from http://www.
fastfoodmarketing.org/media/FastFoodFACTS_Report_2010.pdf.

Wartella, E., and N. Jennings. 2001. Hazards and possibilities of commercial TV
in the schools. In *Handbook of children and the media*, ed. D. G. Singer and J.
L. Singer, 557–70. Thousand Oaks, CA: Sage Publications.

7

STRATEGIES TO WORK COLLABORATIVELY TO PREVENT AN OBESITY EPIDEMIC

LEARNING OBJECTIVES

1. What are some of the evidence-based strategies to collaborate in partnership with home, schools, and stakeholders across the community?
2. How can home, school, and community collaborate for the benefit of children?
3. How can children attain overall healthy development in all domains: physically, cognitively, socially, and emotionally?

"The number of overweight children in America has more than doubled in less than 20 years" (Scully, Barbour, & Roberts-King, 2015). Researching evidence-based strategies to collaborate in partnership with the home environment, schools, and stakeholders across the community, it could be stated that parents, teachers, nurses, and communities need to work together to help promote healthy eating lifestyles in order to help decrease the obesity epidemic.

Communities should require physical education in all schools. The National Association for Sport and Physical Education

(NASPE) and the American Heart Association (AHA) recommend that all elementary school students should participate in 150 minutes per week of PE and that all middle and high school students should participate in 225 minutes of PE per week for the entire school year.

Evidence shows how important movement activities are to children's health; therefore, it is essential for schools to implement multiple physical education classes into the curriculum. Physical education is effective in increasing levels of physical activity and improving physical fitness among children.

Children spend much of their day in school or childcare facilities; therefore, it is important that they are physically active in those settings. Students should be given opportunities for extracurricular physical activity such as physical education classes and outdoor play.

It is a simpler task to instill healthy practices in children when they are young than when they mature into adults. Young children are still learning, while adults become set in their ways. Since children and youth spend so much time in school, childcare providers play a valuable role in encouraging healthy lifestyles. Healthy kids also perform better academically. This is why schools, parents, and communities must unite to inspire youth to make healthy decisions.

There are many factors that contribute to the way a child eats and what they eat. Some of these influences include fast-food restaurants, access to unhealthy snacks in social settings, sugary drinks, and processed food.

Nursingworld.org lists several approaches that nurses can recommend in order to prevent childhood obesity, such as using "social learning theory in partnering with parents to teach new ways of engaging their children in play that promotes physical activity."

Evidence-based strategies that use the collaborative efforts of home, school, and community include the healthy initiatives that have been implemented in schools across the country, such as the *Let's Move!* campaign started by Michelle Obama. These federal initiatives provide schools with healthy eating guidelines, promote nutritional education in schools for children to apply at home, and encourage communities to provide safe environments in which children can be active.

Doctors and nurses can contribute to these efforts to promote children's healthy lifestyles through motivational techniques that incorporate their medical expertise. In a recent study lead by Dietz, "wellness" behaviors are ways doctors and nurses might suggest changes to lifestyle. Health-care providers can assist families in making behavioral changes that eradicate unhealthy habits and contribute to a healthy well-being.

Medical doctors with experience in counseling about diet and activity changes may be well-suited to this role of advisor for families struggling with obesity. Doctors and nurses can collaborate with parents and schools to control the amount of sedentary behavior, to petition for more healthy-eating promotions in the media, to urge local schools to provide more physical activity during school hours, and to eliminate all unhealthy food options from schools (Barlow & Dietz, 2002).

An article on obesity prevention (Davis et al., 2013) discusses a program called CHILE which stands for the "Child Health Initiative for Lifelong Eating and Exercise." The aim of this program is to use a "socioecological approach to improve dietary intake and increase physical activity. . . . The intervention includes: a classroom curriculum; teacher and foodservice training; family engagement; grocery store participation; and healthcare provider support." Teachers and parents receive training on proper nutrition and eating habits, cooks are authorized to change menus, families are invited to various events, and grocery stores provide coupons for healthy items at these events. The researchers found that the implementation of CHILE was both straightforward and effective. This holistic approach involves the family, the school, and the entire community.

An early childhood pilot program called CATCH (Coordinated Approach To Child Health) has been implemented in preschool, creating a nutrition and physical activity curriculum. CATCH is developed into four groupings: classroom curriculum, physical activity, parent education, and teacher training. The result of the carefully thought-out material includes educational standards that are required in preschool using nutritional information as its tool to educate young children. At school, all subject matter can be implemented into the topic of nutrition (Sharma, Chuang, & Hedberg, 2011).

The National Heart Savers Association of Omaha, Nebraska, has implemented a health curriculum for kindergarten through eighth grade to help teachers integrate health and nutrition into classroom lessons. They have laid out an in-depth grade-by-grade breakdown of the values to address and different activities to incorporate into academic learning and physical education.

Activities include a word scramble with fruits as the words or using pulse-taking to learn mathematics. Math, science, social studies, and language arts can easily be incorporated into a nutrition curriculum using these subjects to introduce the information you would like to have students learn on health. Any subject matter can incorporate nutrition at any grade level (National Heart Savers Association, 1999).

The Whole School, Whole Community, Whole Child (WSCC) model expands on the eight elements of the CDC's coordinated school health (CSH) approach and is combined with the whole child framework (Centers for Disease Control and Prevention, 2015). The education, public health, and school health sectors have each called for greater alignment, integration, and collaboration between education and health to improve each child's cognitive, physical, social, and emotional development.

Public health and education serve the same children, often in the same settings. The WSCC focuses on the child to align the common goals of both sectors. The expanded model integrates the eight components of a coordinated school health (CSH) program with the tenets of a whole child approach to education (Centers for Disease Control and Prevention, 2015).

In contrast to evidence-based strategies for other significant health issues, such as tobacco use, the data available regarding the effectiveness of intervention strategies to prevent obesity within communities is still incomplete (Ockene et al., 2007). Both the US Preventive Services Task Force (USPSTF), sponsored by the Agency for Healthcare Research and Quality (AHRQ), and the Community Task Force (CTF), sponsored by the Centers for Disease Control and Prevention, have issued recommendations based on evidence of the effectiveness of options in obesity prevention and promotion of weight loss in primary care and community settings.

Through systematic review of the available research, the CTF recommends the use of interventions aimed at reducing the time children spend viewing TV and other screen media to help control obesity. Such interventions are developed to reduce recreational (that is, neither school-related nor work-related) sedentary screen time and initiate or maintain behavior change. Behavioral screen time interventions are classified into two types:

1. Screen-time-only interventions, which only focus on reducing recreational sedentary screen time.
2. Screen-time-plus interventions, which focus on reducing recreational sedentary screen time and increasing physical activity and/or improving diet.

Both interventions teach behavioral self-management skills through one or more of the following components: classroom-based education, tracking and monitoring, coaching or counseling sessions, and family-based or peer social support.

According to the task force, interventions may also include additional components, such as the use of electronic monitoring devices to limit screen time or setting screen time contingent on physical activity.

COLLABORATION AMONG HOME, SCHOOL, COMMUNITY, AND POLICY MAKERS

It is our duty to make sure that our children grow up happy and healthy. Children mimic the behavior of the adults around them. If we are eating healthy food, our children will eat healthy food. If we are showing them that exercising is fun, they will want to exercise too. We are our child's greatest models for leading a healthy life. It is extremely important to encourage healthy behaviors at home, in school, and throughout the community.

Teachers should continue this trend by allowing students ample gym time and recess time. Teachers can also instruct the students on proper nutrition, and even make meals with them. The community can provide sports leagues, events, cooking classes, and coupons for healthy food in the neighborhood. Policy makers, by promoting healthy advertisements and censoring commercials and media on unhealthy food, can make a huge difference in children's health. Parents will lay the foundation for healthy eating and exercising habits.

The following model could be helpful to all adults who are associated with children and are concerned with children's health.

Proper food and exercise for children is extremely important. There are so many health problems associated with obesity that can be avoided if parents, schools, and communities are committed to making a change. Children who exercise and eat right generally perform better in school, have better self-esteem, and develop healthier relationships with others. Together we can make sure that the rate of childhood obesity drops significantly.

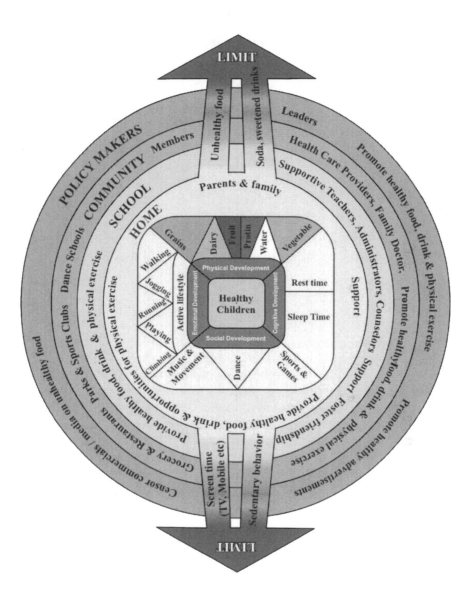

Figure 7.1.   Stay Healthy, Be Happy

"Strategies to Promote the Availability of Affordable Healthy Food and Beverages," from cdc.gov's website, provide helpful tips for collaboration between home, school, and community to help children to grow up healthy. It mentions several strategies that aim to increase the availability of healthy food and beverage choices.

Communities should increase availability of healthier foods and beverages in public venues to ensure that children are not consuming foods and beverages with high sugar, sodium, and fat contents. Schools should aim to provide more nutritious snacks and drinks and meals that offer fruits and vegetables, lower-fat foods, a salad bar, grains, and dairy products.

Communities should provide perks or bonuses, financial or otherwise, to food retailers to locate in underserved areas and to offer healthier food and beverage choices to help improve nutrition and prevent obesity. CDC's website states, "To address this issue, communities can provide incentives to food retailers (e.g., supermarkets, grocery stores, convenience and corner stores, and street vendors) to offer a greater variety of healthier food and beverage choices in underserved areas."

Both options can be offered to "encourage opening new retail outlets in areas with limited shopping options, and existing corner and convenience stores into neighborhood groceries selling healthier foods." Some financial incentives include tax benefits and discounts, loans, and grants to cover start-up and investment costs. Some nonfinancial incentives include supportive zoning.

Another similar model, Epstein's "Model for Parent Involvement" includes: "Parenting, Communicating, Volunteering, Learning at home, Decision-Making and collaboration with the community." All of these points address how important the connection between school, family, community, and home are to child development. All have to work together to provide the best environment for children to learn and develop cognitive, social, emotional, and physical skills, inside and outside of school.

McLeod (2011) in his article, "Bandura's Social Learning Theory (1977)," explains how Albert Bandura believes behavior is learned from the environment through the process of observational learning." According to Bandura's theory, people learn through observing others' behavior and attitudes, and the outcomes of those behaviors.

When parents model positive eating habits, students are able to follow their lead and learn healthy eating habits. Children are products of their environment and some are too young to make choices for themselves so adults must act as guides to show them what foods are good for our bodies and how to stay healthy.

One way to help children learn healthy eating habits is by modeling proper food intake and teaching children the importance of being active. Parents may help support this learning by being active with their children; for example, riding bikes together, going to the park, enrolling children in extracurricular activities. Parents should also remember to pack healthy snacks and water for their children.

Teachers, school nurses, and parents can work together to help formulate a nutritional meal plan for students. According to the article, it is important to "evaluate the readiness of parents to accomplish the lifestyle changes necessary for obesity prevention including their parenting style." All participants need to be active in life. However, children need direction on how to maintain a healthy lifestyle.

Parents should speak with their child's school counselor and nurse so they may have a conversation about behaviors that may contribute to obesity and then collectively list strategies for prevention as well as have them to explain what may be contributing to their child's obesity.

Nurses play a major role in educating parents on how to keep their child healthy and avoid being obese. Nurses help to inform parents about opportunities and strategies for prevention, advise them of steps to take, develop a plan of action, listen to the parents' responses, and reflect on related outcomes and challenges. Schools should work with teachers to help provide nutritious snacks for students and educate parents on healthy meal plans for students.

Further, nutrition policies to tackle childhood obesity need to promote healthy growth and household nutrition security and protect children from inducements to be inactive or to over-consume foods of poor nutritional quality. Toward this goal, family-centered community programs can be appropriate for parents and children, giving them a chance to socialize with peers who are also working to manage their weight.

In addition, schools and communities should ensure that the snacks sold at school canteens are appropriate for a healthy and balanced diet. Parents should also participate actively in preparing a balanced breakfast for their children, as children who eat breakfast get involved in the process of selecting a more balanced diet during the day and have a much smaller percentage of obesity.

Also, a good breakfast is a very important factor in increasing efficiency in school, as concentration and alertness levels are higher. Further, healthy snacks prepared from home can significantly reduce the consumption of food rich in saturated fat and simple carbohydrates. By spending a small portion of their time in such preparations, parents could prevent and treat many of the painful consequences caused by obesity, thus improving the lives of their children.

Such a simple family plan could help to develop eating habits in children that might prevent eating disorders and offer them a healthier and balanced life by reducing the threat posed by obesity to both their physical and mental health.

There are several foods rich in nutrients for children in the earliest years. Among these is extra virgin olive oil, which contains important antioxidants. Known for their antioxidant capacity containing vitamin B, folic acid, and vitamin C, eating green vegetables enhances brain function by maintaining clarity of thought and reducing fatigue. Nuts such as hazelnuts, walnuts, and almonds are a favorite snack for children; they are rich in protein and vitamin E, which is necessary for the development of cognitive skills. As a snack, they are delicious, hearty, and replenish energy and increase alertness in the brain. Grapes and apples are a rich source of flavonoids and antioxidants that boost sound and rapid brain function. Fruits make the mind alert, increase clarity, and give energy and vitality.

Oily fish is a beneficial food for children, because its protein enhances thinking, promotes brain health, memory, concentration ability, and energy. Fish such as salmon, sardines, and tuna are rich in good fats, namely omega-3 fatty acids.

Tomatoes are rich in vitamin E, vitamin B6, minerals, magnesium, phosphorus, lycopene, and many other nutrients that are necessary for the development of a child's immune system to protect against viruses and seasonal influenza.

Chocolates are beneficial to health. They have flavonoids and antioxidants that promote proper brain function. For children it is an extra source of energy to meet the demands of school days. An occasional dark chocolate bar can be a delicious snack for children. Caffeine keeps the brain alert but should not be consumed on a regular basis.

Water helps to hydrate the body and therefore leads to better functioning of the brain. Children should always have a bottle of water with them at school. Schools should allow children to consume water at all times as needed, even while classes are in session.

The nutrients from healthy eating are transformed into the building blocks underlying the composition of the body, while a portion of the food provides the energy for the processes of integration. For these reasons proper nutrition is very important to keep our children healthy. Specifically recommended:

- Increase consumption of fruits and vegetables and whole grains, legumes, and nuts.
- Restrict saturated animal fat and replace it with monounsaturated (olive oil) and polyunsaturated fats, with emphasis on

increasing omega-3 fats (walnuts, hazelnuts, free-range eggs, wild greens, sardines).

- Limit consumption of sugar (trade juices, soft drinks, sweets).
- Reduce fat content, sugar, and salt in processed food.
- Increase physical activity (at least 60 minutes of regular, moderate to vigorous exercise per day).

Parents should reward children with praise rather than with food. Adults should serve food in smaller portions. Let the child ask for more if he or she is still hungry. Snacks should provide nutrients and energy which are essential for active, growing children. Do not give your child vitamin supplements unless they are recommended by your doctor. Keep a variety of snacks in the house, such as fresh fruit, vegetables, whole-grain cereals and crackers. Try lower-calorie or lower-fat foods like baked chips, reduced-sugar cereals, or low-fat dressings.

If poor eating habits are typical and normal at home, it can be hard to change old routines. However, by keeping unhealthy food out of the home and bringing healthy foods in, it's possible to promote healthy habits, even with the pickiest kids. If parents want to buy a treat or a kind of junk food and bring it into the home, buy the smallest possible package of that food instead of the economy, bulk-sized packages.

Encourage kids to drink zero-calorie beverages instead of sugary juices and soda. When cooking dinner, always make sure to have one item that the kid likes and will eat. It is also better to cook extras of the fruits and vegetables to encourage seconds.

Regular physical activity in your daily routine is very important. Try to get between 30 and 60 minutes of physical activity every day (healthychildren.org). Walking as a family before or after meals is a good way to encourage your children to be more active. Increase household activities like walking the dog, dusting, vacuuming, gardening. These activities are good ways to burn calories.

Make playtime with your family more active by playing basketball or walking to the park when it gets warmer. These activities can be a fun way to exercise and establish a good relationship with your children.

Since an overweight child has a higher risk of being bullied, parents should monitor their child in an activity outside of school so that the child can form a new peer group and can develop positive self-esteem. Signing children up for classes at the YMCA or in the neighborhood or joining the Boy or Girl Scouts can be an excellent catalyst for this kind of growth. It is important for parents to help maintain the child's self-esteem by demonstrating respect and acceptance and conveying the message, "I believe in you."

Healthy development in all domains including physical, cognitive, and emotional are important for a child. According to Kids' Nutrition, there are some great exercises to engage in as a class. One example is going on a community walk. The teacher can pick certain things they are supposed to look for on their walk.

Another example is to visit a community store like a grocery store. At the store, a scavenger hunt can be done or teachers can make up different activities. For social and emotional development, children can do a "show and tell" with their favorite foods. At the end of everyone sharing, the class can make their own fruit salad.

Obesity is a serious issue for young children. Since we now know how serious this is, we can move forward to work together as a team to make positive changes. A child's home environment and school environment are such large contributors to a child's lifelong health. Influential environments such as these must work together to create some type of partnership among parents, teachers, and community leaders in order for positive changes to be made.

STRATEGIES FOR HOW SCHOOL AND FAMILY CAN PROMOTE HEALTH AND NUTRITION AMONG CHILDREN AND PREVENT OBESITY

As teachers and parents, we have the responsibility to educate our students on how to independently make well-informed decisions in all aspects of life. Students need to learn how to care for their bodies and their minds. There is a huge difference between teaching children about health and nutrition and the importance of physical exercise and getting them to change their behavior and attitudes, especially when the influence of friends, media, and the environment in which they live and the family experiences and preferences are strong.

Being healthy impacts an individual's everyday life. According to Comer et al. (1996), "When you commit to healthy eating, it means more than choosing fresh veggies over French fries." Children depend on home and school to support them in their well-being and to promote their positive development. Positive reinforcement plays a significant role which can motivate children toward healthy behavior. For example, when children eat something healthy, adults should praise them so that they feel appreciated and are motivated to select healthy food more often. Eating healthy becomes a habit when reinforced regularly.

Another strategy is to invite children to read books about nutrition and exercise. There are books about where food comes from, who grows it, and what kinds of foods are healthy and not so healthy. Children usually like books with illustrations. Teachers can encourage children to evaluate their food choices and also physical activity habits.

After discussing the food pyramid or MyPlate diagrams, teachers should encourage children to make their own diagrams with cutout pictures of food. Teachers can include lunch or snack suggestions in a handbook for parents. Teachers can also list the foods like candy, chips, cookies, or soda that are not permitted in school.

Teachers can suggest that parents bring only fruit or yogurt and water. Comments such as "That banana looks delicious!" or "I love spinach!" help to encourage children to eat healthy foods. In a class party, teachers should provide a list of healthy snacks like carrots, apples, grapes, cheese, and whole-wheat crackers.

Provide a healthy activity board where children can create slogans. A chart can be made and a classroom food-tasting party can be celebrated to enjoy healthy food together.

It is evident that adults influence children's food preferences and their willingness to try new and different foods. Making the children's food environment fun can make all the difference when it comes to mealtime or snack time. The experience needs to be enjoyable. As role models, teachers can share the table with the children and eat healthy foods with them. Interesting and engaging mealtime conversations are also important in creating greater food enjoyment.

Adults can talk positively about the food that they are eating and also encourage the children to describe the colors, tastes, and textures of fruits and vegetables. Students might be motivated if characters from the media are showcased showing healthy behaviors. Teachers could display a poster of a role model from the media exhibiting healthy behaviors to inspire the children. Teachers can recognize children's efforts by writing in school newsletters.

Help children find recipes online and then look at the ingredients to determine if they are healthy or not. Children can make their own cookbooks to keep in a library and take the books home, too; this will help children to feel accomplished and proud of themselves as they follow the recipes in their own book. In order to motivate children, teachers and parents must educate children on the negative effects of unhealthy behavior and inform them about the benefits of a healthy diet and active lifestyle.

Adults need to give children choices in order for them to make independent decisions. Children will be more motivated to make healthy decisions when they are given a choice. The choices should be appealing and accessible. Allow children to have snack options between two healthy items and have a discussion of their selection. Challenge students to eat as many colors of the rainbow as they can in one meal or in one day. Teachers can establish an "Eat your colors" week or month at school and ask parents to send in snacks of the specific color of the week.

Teachers can send home recipe bags filled with healthy and tasty recipes for the student's family to make and enjoy together. At school children could be encouraged to share pictures and discuss their dinner the previous night.

It is a good idea to experiment with dips. Children who do not like to eat vegetables may like to experiment with dips such as hummus, salsa, ranch salad dressing, and yogurt-based dressing. Sometimes a creative way to invite children to eat healthy foods is to address broccoli as "baby trees" or make smiley-face pancakes. Utilizing creativity while making food dishes can be inviting for children. For example, use slices of banana as wheels, pretzel sticks as a wagon, and make a person out of carrot sticks for fun. These creative techniques will help children to enjoy healthy food.

Allowing well-balanced meals three times a day for children will help them grow and establish good eating habits. Help develop healthy eating habits, provide fruits, vegetables, and dairy products, drink ample amounts of water, offer healthy foods during special events, and provide healthy snacks. Involve children on a trip to the supermarket, involve children in cooking activities, create a class-room garden or a school garden, and show them the difference between healthy and unhealthy food items.

Helping students to be more active during recess and after school can motivate children to eat healthier while gaining confidence from participating in sports or extracurricular activities. Teachers can sing songs about healthy eating.

Encourage physical activity at school, during school, and after school, including during recess and in class time. Allow time for dance, yoga, music, movement, and kinesthetic activities. Activities which require active movement as "Simon says" or "duck duck goose" can be used to teach children how to enjoy active movements.

Encourage physical activity at home, limiting sedentary time like TV watching, video games, and computer time. Provide opportunities that require movement. Family activities like playing ping pong, jumping rope, doing yoga, biking, jogging, playing badminton or going swimming could be a good start. Get children to engage in strength-building exercises such as push-ups or sit-ups. Explain to the children how strength-building exercises are important to bone health.

During transition time, between two subject areas, encourage children to do exercises that are fun, for example, do "let's do twenty jumping jacks or toe-touchers." Simple exercise could be reenergizing for the children.

It is important to send a positive message to the students by making healthy eating fun. This positive approach promotes good self-image. Adults are role models. To inspire children, adults can show a popular athlete's healthy eating habits. Kids see adults trying to eat right and getting physically active. It is important to keep things positive. Praise for a job done well and celebrating success helps children develop good self-image.

However, it is important to select true rewards. Food should not be used as a reward; never should children be rewarded with extra hours of TV watching, video games, candy, or unhealthy snacks for a job done well. Adults have to find positive ways to celebrate good behavior, such as going out to the playground for an extra hour or presenting a book as a gift.

Ideally it is better to get the whole family moving. For example, gardening not only motivates children but also raises awareness of the environment. It is important to encourage physical activities that they enjoy so that exercise becomes fun and they look forward to it. Let children explore different activities until they find the exercise they really like.

Limiting screen time (TV, video games, or computer) is essential. Besides being strenuous on the eyes, these habits lead to excessive snacking which increases risks of obesity. Setting realistic goals and limits are key to adopting new behaviors. Small steps and gradual changes can make a big difference in becoming health conscious.

Make dinnertime a family time. When everyone sits down and eats together, there is less chance of children selecting the wrong kinds of food or snacking too much. Adults can monitor children's eating habits and guide them. Further, children should be involved in planning meals and cooking with the family. Make a game of reading food labels. The whole family will learn what is good for their health and be more conscious of what they eat. It is a habit that helps change behavior for a lifetime.

Overall, there are four main reasons for the increase in childhood obesity: an increase in soda consumption, an unhealthy decrease in fruit and vegetable consumption, a decrease in overall physical activity in school, and an increase in sedentary activities (TV, video games, computer usage).

In addition to increasing physical activity, an important step for better weight management is to reduce sedentary activities. It is proven that watching TV is a passive activity that strengthens the sedentary lifestyle and correlates strongly with increasing body weight. In combination with eating junk foods, it exponentially increases the risk of excess weight. Video games and excessive use of computers and mobile phones are also associated with an increased risk of obesity.

Therefore, a reduction in the amount of time spent watching the screen is advised. Sleeping long enough and better scheduling to manage healthier routines will have an immediate impact and benefit on the child's health, especially when combined with increased physical activity. In summary, participation in sports, an increase in general physical activity, and limiting screen time are three important elements which parents can use to enhance the lives of their children and better control their body weight.

DISCUSSION QUESTIONS

1. What are some of the evidence-based strategies to collaborate in partnership with the home, schools, and stakeholders across community?
2. How can home, school, and community collaborate for the benefit of children?
3. How can children attain an overall healthy development in all domains: physically, cognitively, socially, and emotionally?

REFERENCES

Bandura, A. 1977. Social learning theory . Englewood Cliffs, NJ: Prentice Hall.

Barlow, S., and W. Dietz. 2002. Management of child and adolescent obesity: Summary and recommendations based on reports from pediatricians, pediatric nurse practitioners, and registered dietitians. *American Academy of Pediatrics* 110 (1 Suppl) (July). Retrieved from http://pediatrics.aappublications.org/content/110/Supplement_1/236.

Comer, J. P., N. M. Haynes, E. T. Joyner, and M. Ben-Avie, eds. 1996. *Rallying the whole village.* New York: Teachers College Press.

Davis, S. M., S. G. Sanders, C. A. FitzGerald, P. C. Keane, G. F. Canaca, and R. Volker-Rector. 2013. An evidence-based preschool intervention for obesity prevention in Head Start. *Journal of School Health* 83 (3): 223–29.

Dietz, W. H. 1998. Health consequences of obesity in youth: Childhood predictors of adult disease. *Pediatrics* 101 (3 pt 2) (March): 518–25. Retrieved from https://www.ncbi.nlm.nih.gov/pubmed/12224658.

Epstein, J. L., M. G. Sanders, B. S. Simon, K. C. Salinas, N. R. Jansorn, N. Rodriguez, and F. L. Van Voorhis, Corwin. 2002. *School, family, and community partnerships: Your handbook for action*, 2nd edition. Thousand Oaks, CA: Sage.

McLeod, S. A. 2011. Bandura—Social learning theory. *Simply Psychology*. Retrieved from http://www.simplypsychology.org/bandura.html.

Ockene, J. K., E. A. Edgerton, S. M. Teutsch, L. N. Marion, T. Miller, J. L. Genevro, C. J. Loveland-Cherry, J. E. Fielding, and P. A. Briss. 2007. Integrating evidence-based clinical and community strategies to improve health. *American Journal of Preventive Medicine* 32 (3): 244–52.

Scully, P., C. Barbour, and H. Roberts-King. 2015. *Families, schools, and communities: Building partnerships for educating children*, 6th edition. Pearson.

Sharma, S., R. Chuang, & A. M. Hedberg. 2011. Pilot-testing CATCH early childhood: A preschool-based healthy nutrition and physical activity program. *American Journal of Health Education* 42 (1): 12–23.

WEBSITES

http://www.reportingonhealth.org/users/megan

http://www.healthychildren.org

American Heart Association (AHA), http://www.heart.org/HEARTORG/

The National Association for Sport and Physical Education (NASPE), http://www.shapeamerica.org/

Let's Move! https://letsmove.obamawhitehouse.archives.gov/

US Preventive Services Task Force (USPSTF), https://www.uspreventive servicestaskforce.org/

The Community Guide/Community Preventive Services Task Force, https://www.thecommunityguide.org/task-force/community-preventive-services-task-force-members

Centers for Disease Control and Prevention, https://www.cdc.gov/

Whole School, Whole Community, Whole Child (WSCC), http://www.ascd.org/programs/learning-and-health/wscc-model.aspx

Coordinated School Health (CSH), http://www.sparkpe.org/blog/the-eight-components-of-coordinated-school-health/

APPENDIX A

Form for Identifying Risk and Appropriate Interventions

This form can be used as a guide for identifying a child or adolescent at risk for the development of obesity and age appropriate interventions for the child and family.

I. Identification of Risk

A. Anthropometric Risk Factors:

___ parents heights

___ parents weights

___ parents BMIs (>28=overweight)
BMI=(Wgt in lbs/2.2)/(hgt in inches x 0.0254)[2]

B. Feeding Practice Risk Factors:

1. Infants:

___ overfeeding

___ introduction of juice at less than 6 months of age

___ drinking juice from bottles or lidded transportable cups throughout the day

___ limited fruit/vegetable preferences

___ none

2. Toddler:

___ poor fruit and vegetable intake

___ limited fruit and vegetable preferences

___ increased juice or sweetened beverage consumption(>6 oz/day)

___ very fast eater

___ excessive fast food intake

___ controlling feeding practices by caretaker

___ none

3. School-aged Child:

___ poor fruit and vegetable intake

___ increased juice or sweetened beverage consumption(>12 oz/day)

___ very fast eater

___ controlling feeding practices by caretaker

___ excessive fast food intake

___ none

4. Adolescent:

___ increased juice or sweetened beverage consumption (>12 oz/day)

___ poor fruit and vegetable intake

___ very fast eater

___ parents are chronic dieters

___ excessive fast food intake

___ none

C. Activity Pattern Risk Factors:

___ excessive television viewing (>2 hr)

___ sedentary activities

___ limited exercise opportunities

___ none

D. Child's Anthropometric Risk:

Anthropometrics:

___ weight/height plotted on growth charts >85%

___ BMI percentile >85%

___ none

II. Age-appropriate Interventions

Infant:

___ promote breastfeeding

___ counsel to avoid juice prior to 6 months of age

___ encourage water as a between feeding beverage

School-aged Child:

___ healthy snack suggestions

___ slow down when eating (wait 30 min before 2nd portions)

___ Increase water/seltzer

___ decrease TV viewing

___ family activity suggestions

Adolescent:

___ healthy snack suggestions

___ slow down when eating (wait 30 min before second portions)

___ increase water/seltzer

___ decrease TV viewing

___ family activity suggestions

APPENDIX B

Activities for Chapter 2

ACTIVITIES ON NUTRITION UNIT

MYSTERY FOOD BOX

Children will:

- Use their senses to explore healthy food
- Learn about the health benefits of different foods
- Taste fruits and vegetables

Materials:

- An assortment of real fruits and vegetables, whole grains, and low-fat dairy products
- Empty cardboard box (cut a hole in it so children can reach inside)
- Child safety scissors

Ask children: What's your favorite vegetable? Your favorite fruit? When do you drink milk? When do you eat yogurt and cheese?

1. Show children the foods you have brought (for example, fruits and vegetables such as apple, banana, orange, cucumber, broccoli, yucca, bok choy; a small piece of cheese; a whole-wheat pita; an empty yogurt container or a clean, dry low-fat milk carton, etc.) and talk about their colors and shapes. Tell children that this box is a healthy food box.
2. Turn around so the children can't see what you are hiding in the box and place a fruit or vegetable inside the box.
3. Encourage children to take turns reaching inside the box, feeling the food (or its container) inside, and guessing what it is. Ask the child to describe how it feels to the other children. Is it smooth? Bumpy? Is it big or small? What could it be? What makes you think that's what might be inside?
4. Open the box and show the food inside. Discuss the health benefits of each food.

Source: kidshealth.org

VIEW AND DO: I EAT THE COLORS OF THE RAINBOW!

Children will:

- Explore the different colors of fruits and vegetables
- Sort items by colors
- Watch the DVD: "I Eat the Colors of the Rainbow." (Ask children to identify different colors.)

Materials:

- Construction paper (red, orange, yellow, green, blue, and purple)
- Crayons in a variety of colors

- Tape
- Magazines and/or food circulars
- Child safety scissors

Post the colored paper along the wall—red, orange, yellow, green, blue, purple. Make sure it is low to the ground in an area that all children can easily access. Explain that together children will work to create a Healthy Food Rainbow.

Point to a color and ask, "What vegetables or fruits are this color?" Ask children to find pictures to cut out of a magazine or draw a fruit or vegetable. Throughout the week, help children add their healthy food creations to the rainbow wall, posting each one on the color that matches. For example, ask: "Where does broccoli go"? (On the green square)

> Red & Pink: apples, cherries, strawberries, tomatoes, and watermelon
> Yellow & White: bananas, squash, pineapple, corn
> Green: beans, peas, lettuce, grapes, pears, broccoli, spinach
> Orange: oranges, carrots, peaches, cantaloupe, apricot
> Blue & Purple: blueberries, plums, grapes, and eggplant

Then ask the children to gather in front of their beautiful rainbow. What healthy food do they see? All those colors mean so many vitamins and minerals that are good for our bodies.

Source: kidshealth.org

LIFE CYCLE OF A PLANT AND SEED COUNTING

After talking about the growth of an apple tree from seed to tree to apple and back to seed, show the kids an apple and let them guess the number of seeds in it. Then carefully cut open the apple and find out how many there really are. So you don't waste the apple you can have apple slices for snack.

Source: http://www.perfectlypreschool.com

RAINBOW PARFAITS

Materials:

- Plain or vanilla-flavored low fat yogurt
- Colorful cut-up fruit (strawberries, peaches, kiwi, blueberries, bananas, etc.)
- Crushed graham crackers
- Clear plastic cups

In each cup, make layers of yogurt, fruit, and crushed graham crackers.

COLORFUL MENUS

Plan a meal with your child that includes at least three different colors, like red peppers, black beans, and brown rice. Buy the items together. While you're preparing the meal, have your child create a dinner menu or draw a plate with all the food on it. Display the menu near the table, if possible. Have your child count up all the colors on the plate.

NUTRITION UNIT LESSON PLANS

Objective: To help students learn the importance of nutrition in keeping them healthy.

Outline:

Lesson 1: Being Healthy
Lesson 2: Make a Healthy Food Collage
Lesson 3: Food Bingo
Lesson 4: Food Diagram on the Wall
Lesson 5: Colors of Food Posters
Lesson 6: How Do You Differentiate a Fruit from a Vegetable?
Lesson 7: Play Restaurant

LESSON I: BEING HEALTHY

Discussion:

- What can we do to help our bodies stay healthy? (exercise, eat healthy, sleep, brush our teeth, take baths, wash our hands often)
- What kinds of food help to keep us healthy? (fruits, vegetables, meat, eggs, milk)
- Is sleep important for our bodies?
- Should we eat a lot of sweet foods and snacks? Why or why not? (cavities and they are not good for us)
- What is your favorite food to eat?? (pizza, cookies, chicken)
- What is a fruit?
- What is a vegetable?

Read any story about healthy living or healthy foods. Discuss the book. Have posters up in the room with healthy habits on them: for instance children washing their hands, brushing their teeth and eating healthy foods, etc.

LESSON 2: MAKE A HEALTHY FOOD COLLAGE

Objective: To be able to name healthy foods.

Lesson Plan:

Have many food magazines from local grocery stores for children to cut out pictures. Try to have as many colored pictures as possible. The children also need glue, scissors, and a piece of construction paper.

Activity:

- Talk to children about healthy foods.
- Give them each some glue, scissors, and a piece of construction paper. Have them look through the brochures and magazines for pictures of healthy foods they like to eat.
- Then have them cut them out and glue them onto their piece of construction paper.
- When they are all done, they will be able to stand up one at a time in front of the class and tell the other students what they picked out and to point to the picture of that food item.
- Hang them up around the room for parents and other teachers to see.

LESSON 3: FOOD BINGO

Objectives: To learn how to play Bingo and to learn the names of many different kinds of fruits and vegetables.

Lesson Plan:

- Before the day of the lesson, cut out pictures of many different kinds of fruits and vegetables from magazines and glue them onto a piece of construction paper to make a Bingo card. Make enough cards for the number of children in your class.

If possible have these cards laminated so you can use them often.

- Then make up cards with names of all the fruits and vegetables you used on your Bingo cards for the caller to call out. When a child gets three or four in a row, they call Bingo.
- The kids really enjoy this and they can learn new fruits or vegetables if you include pictures of unusual fruits or vegetables such as eggplant and kiwi.

LESSON 4: MYPLATE DIAGRAM

Objectives: To learn about the MyPlate diagram of the food groups and the different sections of it. Also for the children to learn what foods they should have the most to keep them healthy.

Lesson Plan:

- Have a copy of the new MyPlate diagram shape on a wall.
- Leave the plate sections blank for the children to put in the food items. Have a piece of paper in each section that names that part of the plate such as breads.
- Talk to the children about what the plate represents and what each section is.
- Get out pictures of foods and have the children try to put the food in the correct section of the plate.
- After they are done, let them look at what they made and go through the whole MyPlate diagram together as a class, talking about all the examples in each section.
- Also talk about food portions and servings and how much of each serving they are to have a day.

LESSON 5: COLORS OF FOOD POSTERS

Objective: To learn the different colors of foods and make a poster of the different colors to hang on the wall.

Lesson Plan:

- Have many food magazines with many pictures of different colors of food.
- Have four to five pieces of large poster board to glue the pictures onto.
- Label the posters by the color of the food that will be put on it, such as Green Foods, Red Foods, etc.
- After the children cut out the pictures, label each item under the picture, such as tomato, grapes etc.
- After you are all done gluing and making the posters have the children point to an item and the rest of the class tells what it is and what color it is.

The kids loved doing this and looked at the posters often in the room. The posters can be laminated to last longer.

LESSON 6: HOW DO YOU DIFFERENTIATE A FRUIT FROM A VEGETABLE?

Recommended Resource: Fruit & Veggie Sort Learning Center
Objective: To learn the difference between a vegetable and a fruit.

How do you know a vegetable from a fruit? Generally speaking, a fruit is the seed-bearing part of a plant. A vegetable is ANY part of a plant that you would eat (root, stem, leaves, fruit, seeds.)
To dig a bit deeper show the children
Fruit:

- the developed ovary of a seed plant with its contents and accessory parts, such as the pea pod, nut, tomato, or pineapple.
- the edible part of a plant developed from a flower, with any accessory tissues, such as the peach, mulberry, or banana.

Vegetable:

- any plant whose fruit, seeds, roots, tubers, bulbs, stems, leaves, or flower parts are used as food, as the tomato, bean, beet, potato, onion, asparagus, spinach, or cauliflower.
- the edible part of such a plant, as the tuber of the potato.

You may notice tomato was listed as both a vegetable AND fruit.

Bring in some real foods and determine if they are a fruit or a vegetable. Have such examples as corn, tomatoes, green beans, pears, peaches, grapes, etc. Then have them all for a great healthy snack. Have some unusual ones such as kiwi and eggplant if you can find them at your local store.

LESSON 7: PLAY RESTAURANT

Objective: To play restaurant and choose healthy foods when eating out.

Lesson Plan:

- Collect takeout menus from neighborhood restaurants.
- Make menus by drawing pictures of vegetables and dinners and determine the prices of each item.
- Under each picture, put the name of the item and the prices.
- Set up a kitchen area and lots of play food to use to make dinners in their restaurant. Have the students set the table with a plate, cup, and napkin.
- Have them take turns being the waiter, cook, and customer.

Kids love playing this and have so much fun.

Integrating health in subjects throughout the curriculum can be fun and easy! Health does not need to be spoken about in just health and science class, instead it can be discussed in all course subjects. A healthy lifestyle lesson should be taught every week by teachers, especially for young children. It is crucial for them to know about what is good for our bodies, what isn't, and how beneficial being healthy really is.

There are many ways that families can get involved in helping children get the nutritional education they deserve. Parents can play numerous games that are interesting to children and have fun while eating healthy. One activity is called "Make a Rainbow on Your Plate." This is an activity that introduces children to the concept of eating a variety of vegetables for better health by incorporating different colored vegetables into the diet. Children will be able to use nutrition knowledge skills and strategies to promote a healthy lifestyle.

Parents should speak with their child about the different colored vegetables and how they relate to the rainbow. Each day will represent a different color, meaning each day will represent a different vegetable. For example, parents can use the color red for a tomato, the color orange for carrots, the color yellow for peppers, the color indigo for eggplant, etc. Parents should ensure that their child makes a rainbow with fruits and vegetables on their plate. Days can be mixed around as long as every vegetable gets eaten. Parents could also add more options of vegetables. Parents should encourage their child to eat a rainbow every day since different colored vegetables contain different combinations of nutrients. The more colorful, the better! We need a variety of vegetables for a healthy, balanced diet. Fresh vegetables count toward the seven days of eating the rainbow.

School is another environment for positive health experiences. Many activities and lessons can be sent home by teachers that encourage children to eat healthy at home. Educators as well as parents can create a healthy lifestyle for children.

APPENDIX C

Children's Books about Nutrition

The Amazing Milk Book
Catherine Ross, Paulette Bourgeois, and Susan Wallace
This book describes milk's chemistry, nutritional value, production, and use as a
component of cheese and other food. It's enriched with anecdotes and humor.
The Beastly Feast
Bruce Goldstone
At the great animal feast, bears bring pears and mosquitoes bring burritos.
Belly Laughs!
Charles Keller
These 75 food jokes and illustrations are written especially for children.
Blue's Snack Party
Sarah Landy
Blue's friends bring healthy snacks to a party. Discover each snack by lifting
flaps that reveal ingredients, recipes, and finished dishes.
A Book of Fruit
Barbara Hirsch Lember
While most children recognize fruit in a bowl or in a supermarket, some have
never seen fruit growing on a tree or a bush. This well-photographed book
makes the connection between the fruit and where and how it grows before it
arrives at the supermarket. Photos of single servings of fruit appear on pages
opposite photos of where the fruit grows.
Bread, Bread, Bread
Ann Morris
With large photographs, this book depicts the wide variety of breads from around
the world. From India to Mexico, from Peru to Indonesia, from Ghana to
Greece, international breads are shown.

Bread is for Eating
David and Phillis Gershator
Mamita explains how bread is created and sings, "El pan es para comer" ("Bread Is For Eating"). Music and lyrics in both Spanish and English are included.

Cloudy with a Chance of Meatballs
Judi Barrett
The townspeople love it when food falls from the sky—until the food gets too big to swallow.

Cooking Up U.S. History: Recipes and Research to Share with Children
Suzanne I. Barchers and Patricia C. Marden
This book supplies a word list, recipes, and a bibliography for five historical periods of US history and six regions of the United States.

Dinner at the Panda Palace
Stephanie Calmenson
Babies and toddlers see animals dining out at the Panda Palace.

Dinosaurs Alive and Well; A Guide to Good Health
Laurie Krasny Brown and Marc Brown
Colorful and bright dinosaurs provide kids with a blueprint to good health. Nutrition, exercise, and fitness are some of the topics that are encountered.

Dumpling Soup
Jama Kim Rattigan
A young Hawaiian girl tries to make dumplings for her family's New Year celebration. This story celebrates the joyful mix of food, customs, and languages of many cultures.

D. W. the Picky Eater
Marc Brown
Arthur the Aardvark's sister, D. W., is a picky eater. The family leaves her at home when they go out to eat until D. W. decides she might be missing something good by being so picky.

The Edible Pyramid: Good Eating Every Day
Loreen Leedy
At the Edible Pyramid Restaurant, guests learn about all the foods they can eat from USDA's Food Guide Pyramid.

Everybody Cooks Rice
Norah Dooley
Anthony is late for dinner. So his sister goes from house to house looking for him. In each home, she finds families preparing rice in a different way. This multicultural dinner tale ends with several recipes for rice—from Barbados, Puerto Rico, Vietnam, India, China, Haiti, and Italy.

Extra Cheese, Please!: Mozzarella's Journey from Cow to Pizza
Chris Peterson
This well-photographed book describes how cheese is made, from a Wisconsin dairy farm until a cheese factory ships the final product across America.

Family Pictures: Cuadros de Familia
Carmen Lomas Garza

The author describes, in bilingual text and illustrations, her experiences growing up in a Hispanic community in Texas. Several of the stories focus on food-picking, cactus, making tamales, eating tacos, picking oranges, and eating watermelon.

Foods: Feasts, Cooks, and Kitchens

Richard Tames

This history of food discusses the types of foods and cooking methods used by cultures from the hunters and gatherers of 18,000 BC to Egyptians, Greeks, Romans, Middle Ages, and all the way to futuristic farming. It's filled with interesting illustrations and fascinating facts.

Grandpa's Garden Lunch

Judith Caseley

Take a trip down to the garden with Sarah and her Grandpa and learn the basics of gardening. Kids will learn about how various foods grow. They will also see why "patience is a virtue."

Gregory, The Terrible Eater

Mitchell Sharmat

Gregory the goat likes eggs, vegetables, fruit, and fish. But his parents want him to eat garbage!

Group Soup

Barbara Brenner

A selfish rabbit learns that sharing is the one ingredient needed to make the perfect Group Soup.

How My Family Lives in America

Susan Kuklin

This book tells the story of three children, each with an immigrant parent. For each family, the foods they eat, the names of different dishes, and their eating customs are discussed. The book includes three recipes—one African, one Puerto Rican, and one Taiwanese.

How to Make an Apple Pie and See the World

Marjorie Priceman

Since the supermarket is closed, the reader is led around the world—to Italy, France, Sri Lanka, England, Jamaica, and Vermont—to gather the ingredients for making an apple pie.

I Know an Old Lady Who Swallowed a Pie

Alison Jackson

In this take-off on the song "I Know an Old Lady Who Swallowed a Fly," a woman rudely eats everything at a Thanksgiving feast!

I Will Never Not Ever Eat a Tomato

Lauren Child

Charlie convinces his sister Lola to eat fruits and vegetables. For example, Charlie calls mashed potatoes "cloud fluff from the pointiest peak of Mount Fuji."

It's a Spoon, Not a Shovel

Mark and Caralyn Buehner

When a crocodile is eating an armadillo, should she put her napkin (a) on her head, (b) in her ear, or (c) on her lap? This is a humorous etiquette book for young children.

Macho Nacho and Other Rhyming Riddles
Giulio Maestro
This book is filled with rhyming riddles, many of which are riddles about foods.

Make Me a Peanut Butter Sandwich and a Glass of Milk
Ken Robbins
This book describes the production of three foods: peanut butter, bread, and milk . . . from the farm to the manufacturing plant to the store to the home.

A Medieval Feast
Aliki
A manor prepares a feast fit for a king and queen.

Milk From Cow To Carton
Aliki
Aliki takes readers on a guided tour that begins with grazing cows, proceeds through milking and a trip to the dairy, and ends with some different foods made from milk.

Multicultural Cookbook for Students
Carole L. Allyn and Lois S. Webb
This cookbook includes 337 recipes from 122 countries. Also included are maps and background information about each country. The ingredients on the recipes are food generally available in the United States.

Munching: Poems about Eating
Selected by Lee Bennett Hopkins
A collection of over 20 poems about food for children.

Never Take a Pig to Lunch and Other Poems about the Fun of Eating
Selected and illustrated by Nadine Bernard Westcott
A collection of 50 poems and traditional rhymes about food and eating.

No Milk!
Jennifer Ericsson
A city boy tries to coax, cajole, coerce, and command the milk out of a dairy cow—but no milk! As tempers flare, the pair finally arrives at a creamy compromise. Perfect for reading aloud.

Pass the Fritters, Critters
Cheryl Chapman
Should the bunny pass the honey? Should the parrot pass the carrots? Not without the magic word!

Peanut Butter, Apple Butter, Cinnamon Toast: Food Riddles for You to Guess
Argentina Palacios
A book of food riddles for children.

Pizza!
Teresa Martino
A brief history of pizza for beginning readers.

The Race Against Junk Food

Anthony Buono

Tommy and the Snak Posse (which includes vegetable-people) win a footrace against junk food.

Roses Sing on New Snow

Paul Yee

Set in turn-of-the-century Chinatown, this is the story of a young girl who cooks in her father's restaurant. Although her father never gives Maylin credit for her great cooking, she works hard because she loves food and loves preparing meals for Chinese immigrants away from their families. When her father presents her new dish to the governor of South China, the truth comes out and Maylin is finally recognized as a very special cook.

A Spoon for Every Bite

Joe Hayes

A poor Southwestern couple buys a third spoon so they can invite their baby's godfather to dinner. Their rich guest brags about his numerous spoons, so the couple tells a story about someone who uses a new spoon for every bite. What they're really referring to is a tortilla, but the rich man is fooled and buys spoons until he's broke.

The Tawny, Scrawny Lion

Kathryn Jackson

A rabbit avoids being eaten by a lion by serving him delicious carrot stew.

This Is the Way We Eat Our Lunch

Edith Baer and Steve Björkman

Kids are taken around the world to learn about the various lunch preferences of children from different cultures. Colorful illustrations help make this adventure to various destinations extra special.

Too Many Tamales

Gary Soto

While helping make tamales for Christmas dinner, Maria tries on her mother's ring. When she realizes the ring is missing, her cousins come to the rescue.

The Vegetable Show

Laura Krasny Brown

Watch vegetables do a little vaudeville in their attempt to dance and sing their way onto the plates and into the hearts of kids. Kids will truly be tempted by the delightful characters including the Tip-Top Tomato Twins and Bud the Spud.

The Victory Garden Vegetable Alphabet Book

Jerry Pallotta and Bob Thomson

This book depicts a vegetable for each letter of the alphabet. The art and text help students to make important associations between vegetables and other familiar things in the environment.

What Am I? Looking Through Shapes at Apples and Grapes

Diane and Leo Dillon

Invite children to guess each food described in a rhyme and shown through a hole on the right-hand page. Turn the page for the answer!

What Food Is This?

Rosmarie Hausherr

Fish, sausage, carrots, and many more foods are detailed in this tale of food
origins. Kids can tune up their food trivia skills as they are quizzed with
questions and pictures. This book is educational as well as fun for the whole
family.

APPENDIX D

Additional Books, Websites, and Other Resources

BOOKS

A Big Cheese for the White House, Candace Fleming, 978-0374406271
A Beekeeper's Year, Sylvia A. Johnson, 0-316-46745-6
A Passion for Proteins, Kristin Petrie, 1-59197-405-4
Apples, Gail Gibbons, 978-0-8234-1669-0
Bread, Bread, Bread, Ann Morris, 0-688-12275-2
Burp! The Most Interesting Book You'll Ever Read About Eating, Diane Swanson, 978-1550746013
Corn Is Maize, Aliki, 0-06-445026-0
Dairy, Susan Derkazarian, 0-516-25925-3
Dinner Time! Dawn Sirett, 978-0-7566-2583-2
Eat Healthy, Feel Great, Martha Sears, 978-0316787086
Eating the Alphabet, Lois Ehlert, 0-15-224436-0
Food Rules! The Stuff You Munch, Its Crunch, Its Punch, and Why You Sometimes Lose Your Lunch, Bill Haduch, 978-0141311470
From Cow to Ice Cream, Bertram T. Knight, 0-516-26066-9
From Wheat to Pasta, Robert Egan, 0-516-26069-3
Garden Partners, Diane Palmisciano, 978-0689314155
Goldilocks and the Three Bears, James Marshall, 0-14-056366-0
Good Enough to Eat, Lizzy Rockwell, 978-0064451741
Grains to Bread, Inez Snyder, 0-516-25527-4
Gregory, the Terrible Eater, Mitchell Sharmat, 978-0545129312
Group Soup, Barbara Brenner, 978-0670828678
Growing Vegetable Soup, Lois Ehlert, 0-15-232580-8
Harvest Year, Cris Peterson, 978-1590787830

Healthy Eating with My Pyramid, Mari C. Schuh, 978-0-7368-6925-6
Herb, the Vegetarian Dragon, Jules Bass and Debbie Harter, 978-1905236473
How a Seed Grows, Helene Jordan, 13:978-0-06-445107-9
How Do Apples Grow? Betsy Maestro, 0-06-445117-8
How to Teach Nutrition to Kids, Connie Liakos Evers, 978-0964797017
I Will Never NOT EVER Eat a Tomato, Lauren Child, 978-0763621803
If You Give a Mouse a Cookie, Laura Joffe Numeroff, 0-06-024587-5
Janice VanCleave's Food and Nutrition for Every Kid, Janice VanCleave, 978-0471176657
Johnny Appleseed, Steven Kellogg, 978-0688064174
Kiss the Cow, Phyllis Root, 0-7636-2003-3
Little Pea, Amy Krouse Rosenthal, 10-0-8118-4658-X
Lunch, Denise Fleming, 0-8050-4646-1
Meats and Proteins, Robin Nelson, 0-8225-4630-2
Milk: From Cow to Carton, Aliki Brandenberg, 0-06-445111-9
More Spaghetti, I Say! Rita Golden Gelman, 0-590-45783-7
My Food Pyramid, Alisha Niehaus, 978-0-7566-29992-2
Orange Pear Apple Bear, Emily Gravett, 1-4169-3999-7
Oliver's Fruit Salad, Vivian French, 978-0340704530
Pancakes for Breakfast, Tomie dePaola, 0-15-670768-3
Peas and Thank You, Mike Nawrocki, 0-15-670768-3
Popcorn, Millicent E. Selsam, 0-688-22083-5
Protein, Justine and Ron Fontes, 0-516-24650-X
Red Red Red, Valerie Gorbachev, 978-0399246289
Seeds and More Seeds, Millicent Selsam, 978-0060253950
Showdown at the Food Pyramid, Rex Barron, 978-0-399-23715-7
Silly Snacks: Cooking with Kids, Sesame Street: Publications International Staff, 978-1412729437
The Big Stew, Ben Shecter, 0-06-025610-9
The Busy Body Book, Lizzy Rockwell, 978-0553113747
The Carrot Seed, Ruth Krauss, 978-0694004928
The Cooking Book, Laura J. Colker, 978-1928896203
The Edible Pyramid, Loreen Leedy, 0-8234-1233-4
The Food Pyramid, Joan Kalbacken, 978-0516263762
The Grain Group, Mari C. Schuh, 978-0736866675
The Healthy Body Cookbook, Joan D'Amico, 978-0471188889
The Hole by the Apple Tree, Nancy Polette, 0-688-10557-2
The Honey Makers, Gail Gibbons, 0-688-11386-9
The Joy of Soy: Vegetarian Cartoons, Vance Lehmkuhl, 978-1889594033
The Little Red Hen, Carol Ottolenghi, 1-57768-378-1
The Meat and Protein Group, Helen Frost, 0-7368-0539-7
The Milk Makers, Gail Gibbons, 0-02-736640-5
The Popcorn Book, Tomie dePaola, 0-8234-0314-9
The Princess and the Pizza, Mary Jane and Herm Auch, 0-8234-1798-8
The Race Against Junk Food, Anthony Buono, 978-0965810807

The Runaway Rice Cake, Ying Chang Compestine, 0-689-82972-8
The Senses, Angela Royston, 0-8120-6272-8
The Spice of Life (Kids' Stuff), Kay Dunbar, 978-0947882198
The Tortilla Factory, Gary Paulsen, 0-15-201698-8
The Very Hungry Caterpillar, Eric Carle, 978-0399226908
Three Stalks of Corn, Leo Politi, 0-684-14572-3
Town Mouse/Country Mouse, Lorinda Bryan Cauley, 0-399-21123-3
Wash Your Hands, Tony Ross, 978-1929132010
We Can Eat the Plants, Rozanne Williams, 0-91619-26-2

WEBSITES

http://www.dole5aday.com
http://www.fruitandveggiesmorematters.org
http://www.dltk-kids.com
http://www.tropicana.com
http://www.everythingpreschool.com
http://www.web.aces.edu/wellnessways
http://www.monroe.k12.fl.us/headstart/Very_Hungry_Catepillar_LP.pdf
http://www.chaquita.com
http://www.kidshealth.org
http://www.msu.edu
http://www.USDA.com
http://www.nutritionexplorations.org
http://www.mypyramid.gov
http://www.dshs.state.tx.us
http://www.healthychoices.org
http://classroom.kidshealth.org/classroom/cc/EveryDayIsAHealthyDay.pdf
http://wholegrainscouncil.org
http://exploratorium.edu/cooking/bread/index.html
http://life.familyeducation.com/foods/nutrition-and-diet/44290.html?detoured=1
http://kidshealth.org/kid/nutrition/food/go_slow_whoa.html
http://www.eduref.org/Virtual/Lessons/Health/Nutrition/NUT0017.html
http://neatsolutions.com/
http://www.3adaysuperfans.org
http://www.freshforkids.com

OTHER RESOURCES

Bales, D., C. Wallinga, and M. Coleman. 2006. Health and safety in the early childhood classroom: Guidelines for curriculum development. *Childhood Education Infancy Through Early Adolescence* 82 (3): 132–38.

The Education Center, Inc. 2001. Goldilocks and the three bears. *The Mailbox: The Idea Magazine for Teachers* (June/July): 16–20.

The Education Center, Inc. 2001. Seed snipe: Apple activity sheet. *The Mailbox: The Idea Magazine for Teachers* (June/July): 20–21.

INDEX

academic achievement, 7; breakfast for, 45, 110; CDC research on health and, 141–142; childhood obesity influencing, 96; exercise supporting, 68–69; nutrition as basis for, 44–46, 45, 50; students, lunch choices and, 48; students and lunch choices as, 48

adiposity rebound, 39, 104

adolescent changes, 81

advertisements, 4, 155; childhood obesity linked to, 86, 148–149, 149; children exploited by, 146, 147, 149; eating disorders contributed by, 86; emotional health influenced by, 86–89; fast food types of, 151–152; on Internet, 150, 155; in schools, 150–152; on television, 146, 149; unhealthy diets result of, 147, 152

asthma, 13, 104

autism, 77

behavior modification, 37–38; breakfast for, 110; childhood obesity prevention in, 14, 28

Bingo, for nutrition education, 188–189

blood pressure, 13

BMI. *See* body mass index

BMI data: on Hispanic and black children, 15–16; on Native American children, 15–16; per CDC, 15

body mass index (BMI), 85; as child obesity measure, 28; exercise resulting in lower, 28, 75, 140; fast food restaurants raising, 14; gardening for lowering, 138; metabolic syndrome predicted by, 14; screen time related to, 15, 178; self-esteem influenced by, 13, 83–84, 84–85, 86, 92, 96; television increasing, 15, 148, 178; weight indicated from childhood, 16–17

brain function, 71; fatty foods creating scars on, 107; iron deficiency reducing, 52, 67; water for hydration and, 171

breakfast, 19, 22; for academic achievement, 45, 110; energy during day from, 109–110; frequency of, 45, 46; gifted students eating, 45, 51–52; quality of, 46, 46–47

bullying: on cell phone or online, 95; childhood obesity as creating, 85, 95; childhood obesity subjected to, 13, 89–93; children responding to, 90–91, 93–94; community responses to, 90, 97; counselor responses to, 90, 93; depression from, 90, 97; exercise as response to, 91; group support as reducing, 93, 94; life-long influences from, 87, 88, 92, 97; parents and teachers informed of, 84, 93, 93–94; peer pressure worsened by, 95; prevention of, 99; responses to, 93–95;

ABOUT THE AUTHOR

Smita Guha is an associate professor in the Department of Curriculum and Instruction in the School of Education at St. John's University, New York. She has been a university faculty for more than twenty years and has over eighteen years of experience working with young children.